Baby & Child
Emergency
First Aid

Simple Step-by-Step Instructions for the
Most Common Childhood Emergencies

Baby & Child Emergency First Aid

Simple Step-by-Step Instructions for the Most Common Childhood Emergencies

Edited by
Mitchell J. Einzig, MD
with **Paula Kelly**, MD

Meadowbrook Press
Distributed by Simon & Schuster
New York

Library of Congress Cataloging-in-Publication Data

Einzig, Mitchell J.
  Baby & child emergency first-aid handbook / by Mitchell J. Einzig. -- [Rev. ed.]
      p. cm.
   title: Baby and child emergency first-aid handbook
   MBP ISBN-13: 978-0-88166-567-3; S&S ISBN-13: 978-1-4391-8646-6
   1. Pediatric emergencies--Handbooks, manuals, etc. 2. First aid in illness and injury--Handbooks, manuals, etc.
I. Title. II. Title: Baby and child emergency first-aid handbook.
   RJ370.B3 2011
   618.92'0025--dc22
                          2010038612

Executive Editor: Megan McGinnis
Creative Director: Tamara JM Peterson
Cover Photos: Amy Segner & Brenna Segner © Meadowbrook Creations, © Ian Hooton, © JGI
Interior Illustrations: Nancy Lynch & Susan Spellman

Text © 2010 Meadowbrook Creations

Although the authors and publisher have made every effort to ensure that the information in this book is accurate and current, only your caregiver knows you and your health history well enough to make specific recommendations. The authors, editors, reviewers, and publisher disclaim any liability from the use of this book.

Published by Meadowbrook Press, 5451 Smetana Drive, Minnetonka, MN 55343

www.meadowbrookpress.com

BOOK TRADE DISTRIBUTION by Simon & Schuster, a division of Simon & Schuster, Inc.
1230 Avenue of the Americas, New York, NY 10020

15 14 13 12 11 10   10 9 8 7 6 5 4 3 2 1

Printed in the United States of America

Call 1-800-338-2232 for a quantity discount.

Contents

Contents

Introduction

As a father and pediatrician, I know that nothing is more frightening than when your child experiences a medical emergency. Other than calling an emergency number, parents are often unsure of what to do. With most emergencies, however, there are steps you can take to help your child before medical help is available. *Baby & Child Emergency First Aid* is designed to provide you with those first-aid steps that sometimes save lives.

Most emergency first-aid books currently available overwhelm you with excessive information that is often impractical and poorly organized. The illustrations in these books often do not clearly relate to the text and may look stark and frightening.

Based on my years of experience in pediatrics, I have selected the most common childhood emergencies and provided you with directions for essential, practical first-aid treatment.

This book is designed to be easily read during an emergency. Use the index on the back cover (or the table of contents) to look up the specific topic you need. On the page indicated, you'll find information required before you begin first aid, including instructions on when to get professional help, which signs and symptoms to monitor, and what *not* to do. The first-aid steps are clearly numbered, written in large type, and accompanied by reassuring illustrations.

When you get this book, first fill out the Parents' Emergency Information Page at the back of the book so the phone numbers you need will be readily at hand. It is also a good idea to have the emergency first-aid supplies listed on page viii. Next, read through the emergency first-aid treatment entries to familiarize yourself with basic information about specific emergencies. Be sure to keep the book in an easily accessible location. Finally, take a basic course in CPR (cardiopulmonary resuscitation) if you have not already done so, or retake it if you have not done so in the last one to two years. The techniques for CPR are most effectively and safely learned and reviewed through personal instruction and supervised practice.

I hope you never have occasion to use this book. But if you do, it will help you take safe, effective action in an emergency until professional help is available. Good luck to you and your family.

Mitchell J. Einzig, M.D.

First-Aid Supplies

Keep the following supplies out of children's reach, but easily accessible in an emergency. You may want to assemble one kit for home and another for your vehicle.

- Adhesive bandages: assorted sizes
- Adhesive tape: ½ to 1 inch (1¼ to 2½ cm) wide
- Antibiotic ointment
- Antihistamines (over-the-counter)
- Antiseptic wipes, towelettes, or solution
- Bulb-suction device or turkey baster, to flush wounds
- Calamine lotion
- Cool-mist vaporizer
- Cold pack, instant
- Cotton balls
- Cotton swabs
- Duct tape
- Elastic bandages
- Eye goggles
- First-aid manual
- Gloves, disposable latex or synthetic
- Heating pad
- Hot-water bottle
- Lubricant/petroleum jelly
- Pain-relieving tablets or liquid (acetaminophen or ibuprofen)
- Plastic bags for disposal of contaminated materials
- Save-A-Tooth container (http://www.save-a-tooth.com)
- Scissors with blunt tips
- Soap
- Sterile eye wash
- Sterile gauze bandages and pads
- Syrup of ipecac
- Thermometer, digital (oral, axillary), temporal artery (TemporalScanner), or rectal
- Triangular bandages and safety pins
- Tweezers (round-ended)

How to Make a Splint

A splint is used to immobilize an injured body part and protect it from further injury. In general, don't try to move or reposition a fractured bone or dislocated joint. Always immobilize it in the position in which it was found. Follow these general steps when splinting a body part.

1. Use something rigid and flat for the splint, such as a board, ruler, stick, or rolled-up magazine or newspaper. You can also use a pillow, blanket, rolled-up piece of clothing, or in some cases another body part, such as a leg or finger.

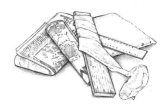

2. If the splint is hard and rigid, pad it with cloths or towels before attaching it.

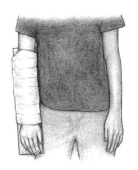

3. Be certain the splint extends to the joints above and below a fracture.

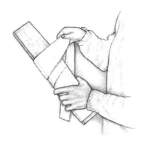

4. Tie the splint to the injured part with cloth strips, tape, belts, or neckties. Be careful not to attach the splint too tightly; if the fingers or toes become pale and cool, loosen the splint. Don't let knots press against the injured area.

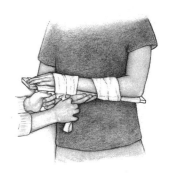

How to Make a Sling

A sling is used to immobilize an injured shoulder, collarbone, or forearm and place it in a position of comfort. Follow these general steps when making a sling.

1. Make a triangular sling by folding a square yard of cloth diagonally, or improvise by using an item of clothing.

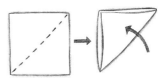

2. Have your child support her injured arm while you slip the sling under the arm, as shown.

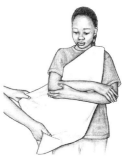

3. Fold the cloth around the arm and pull the edges up over your child's shoulders.

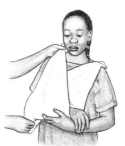

4. Tie a knot on the side of your child's neck. Pin up the extra cloth at her elbow.

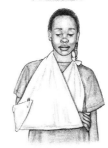

5. With some injuries, to decrease mobility, tie the sling to your child's body with another piece of cloth, knotting the cloth on the uninjured side.

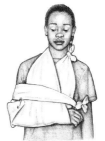

Emergency First-Aid Treatment

Allergic Reactions/Anaphylaxis

What You Need to Know

- An allergy is a sensitivity to a specific substance (e.g., food, drug, insect stings, or latex). Anaphylaxis is an extreme sensitivity to a specific substance.
- The majority of allergic reactions are relatively mild and can be treated at home. An anaphylactic reaction can involve multiple systems, be severe or life threatening, and require medical treatment.
- Most severe reactions occur relatively soon after contact with or ingestion of a foreign substance. (Some reactions can be delayed.)

When to Get Professional Help

- If your child has difficulty breathing, call your local emergency number.
- If you think your child is having an allergic reaction, call your doctor.

Signs & Symptoms

- Rash with or without hives; itchiness; flushed or pale skin; lip, eye, throat, or face swelling; stuffy nose; dizziness; abdominal pain; vomiting; diarrhea; difficulty breathing; wheezing.
- If very severe, shock (clammy skin; rapid, shallow breathing; fainting or becoming unconscious; weak, rapid pulse). For more information, turn to page 79—SHOCK.

1. Calm and reassure your child; anxiety can increase the severity of a reaction.

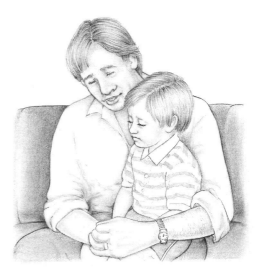

2. If the reaction is mild, give your child over-the-counter antihistamines.

   Check first with your doctor if your child is taking other medication.

   Follow the dosage and age guidelines recommended on the package label.

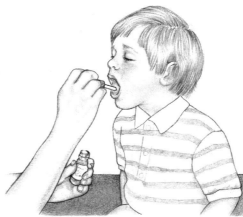

What to Check
- Observe your child's breathing and check the pulse. If needed, begin CPR:

  If your child is under 1 year old, see page 16, BREATHING/CARDIAC EMERGENCY, For Infant Under 1 Year.

  If your child is 1 to 8 years old, see page 20, BREATHING/CARDIAC EMERGENCY, For Child Age 1–8 Years.

  If your child is over 8 years old, see page 24, BREATHING/CARDIAC EMERGENCY, For Child Over 8 Years.

- Look for a medical alert bracelet or necklace and follow the instructions. Or if you can't see an alert tag, if possible ask your child if she is carrying an allergy notification and any allergy medication such as an EpiPen or Twinject device. If so, ask her if she needs your help to use it.

3. If your child has an itchy rash, apply calamine lotion or cool compresses to alleviate itching.

   Do not apply calamine lotion to your child's face or genitals.

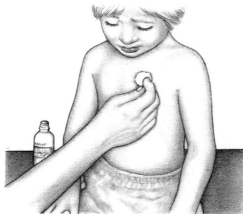

Amputation (Traumatic)

What You Need to Know

- Traumatic amputation is the loss of a body part—usually all or part of a finger, toe, arm, or leg—that occurs from trauma or an accident.
- Remain calm; severed parts often can be surgically reattached. Save even small severed parts.

When to Get Professional Help

- If your child severs a limb, finger, or toe, call your local emergency number immediately.

1. Reassure and comfort your child.

   Assess her ABC (airway, breathing, circulation) and check for the possibility of shock. For more information, turn to page 79—SHOCK.

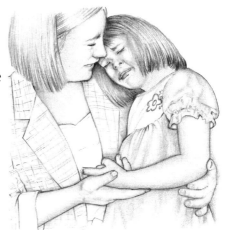

2. If the stump is bleeding, apply direct pressure with a clean, dry cloth.

   Maintain firm but gentle pressure for 5 to 10 minutes or until the bleeding subsides. If blood soaks through the cloth, don't remove it; you may loosen the clot. Place another cloth over the first one.

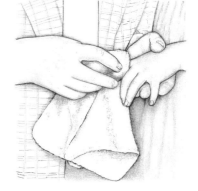

3. When the bleeding has subsided, even if the wound is still oozing, cover the stump with a clean cloth.

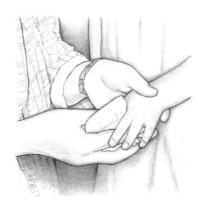

4

4. If possible, raise the injured area above heart level to reduce bleeding.

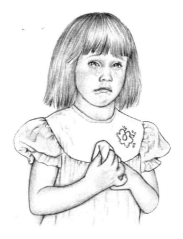

Don'ts
- Don't apply a tourniquet unless the amputation is life threatening.
- Don't attempt to put a severed part back in place.
- Don't forget to check for other injuries.

5. Wrap the severed part in a clean, damp cloth, place it in a sealed plastic bag, and immerse the bag in cold water, preferably ice water. This can help preserve the chance of reattachment up to 18 hours later.

Don't put the severed part directly on ice. If cold water is not available, keep the part away from heat. Save it for the emergency personnel or take it with you to the hospital. Make sure the body part stays with your child.

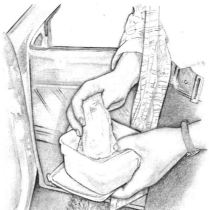

Asthma

What You Need to Know

- Asthma is a chronic disease that is caused by swelling and irritation of the airways. Preventive management of triggers is the best way to avoid asthma episodes.
- Asthma and allergies can overlap, with some asthma events being triggered by allergies.
- Symptoms are often worse at night.

Signs & Symptoms

- Coughing, wheezing, difficulty breathing, aching, or tightness in the chest. Note that coughing and wheezing can disappear because the airway has become too narrow to make noise.
- In severe cases, the symptoms can include sweating, fainting, nausea, panting, a fast pulse, and cold, moist skin.

1. Calm and reassure your child; anxiety can increase the severity of asthma.

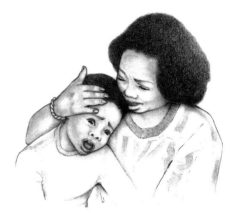

2. Give your child his prescribed medication.

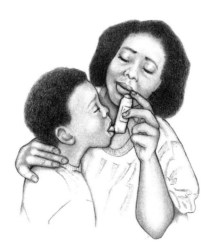

3. Give your child clear liquids.

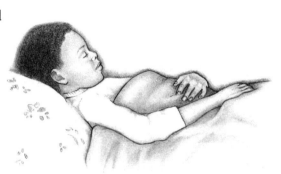

4. Have your child rest in a well-ventilated room.

If he has difficulty breathing while lying down, have him sit up.

When to Get Professional Help

- If your child (a) is experiencing asthma for the first time, (b) does not respond to his prescribed treatment, or (c) has a temperature over 102°F (39°C), call your doctor.
- Call your local emergency number if there are signs of respiratory failure, including shortness of breath even while lying down, blue or gray lips or fingertips, the need to take a breath to complete sentences, agitation or confusion, hunched shoulders, or straining of neck, chest or abdominal muscles.

Bites & Stings

Animal & Human Bites

What You Need to Know

- Puncture wounds—which are common with cat and human bites—pose the highest risk of infection. Human bites can have an equal—or higher—incidence of infection as animal bites. Dog bites have a lower incidence of infection.

When to Get Professional Help

- If your child has multiple bites and/or severe bleeding, or if a bite broke the skin, call your local emergency number.
- If a child is bitten on the face, neck, or hand, or near a joint, call your doctor.

Don't

- Don't clean the bite with alcohol or hydrogen peroxide, which may injure normal tissue.

1. If the bite is bleeding profusely, apply direct pressure with a clean, dry cloth until the bleeding subsides.

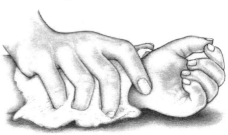

2. Wash the bite thoroughly with soap and lukewarm running water for 3 to 5 minutes and pat dry.

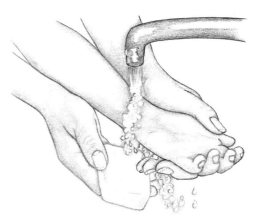

3. Apply antibiotic cream and cover the bite with a clean dressing.

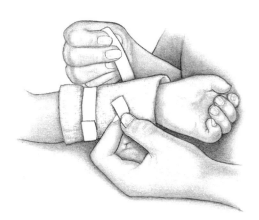

4. Over the next 24 to 48 hours, observe the bite for signs of infection (increasing redness, swelling, oozing, and pain).

If the bite looks infected, call your doctor or take your child to an emergency facility.

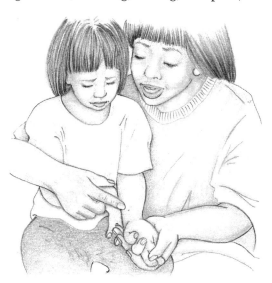

What to Check

- Determine whether your child's vaccinations are current. Tetanus immunity needs to be boosted every 10 years. A deep or dirty wound may require tetanus immunity within the last 5 years. If immunity is not up to date, it is important to get a booster as soon as possible after the injury.
- Observe the animal's behavior. Rabies are a particular concern with bats, skunks (North America only), foxes, raccoons, and stray cats and dogs. Domestic animals of unknown immune status need to evaluated and observed for possible risk. Rabies are rarely a concern with squirrels, rabbits, hamsters, gerbils, and other rodents.

Bites & Stings
Bee Stings & Insect Bites

What You Need to Know
- Bee stings and insect bites occur when there is injection of venom or some other foreign substance into the skin.
- Severe reactions to bee stings are very uncommon and usually occur shortly after the sting. Numerous stings at one time can increase the risk of a severe reaction.

When to Get Professional Help
- If your child has difficulty breathing, call your local emergency number.
- If your child has a rash, call your doctor.

Signs & Symptoms
- A *mild reaction* may include pain, redness, annoying itching and stinging, and 1 to 2 inches (2½ to 5 cm) of swelling around the bite, usually lasting less than 24 to 48 hours.
- A *severe—and possibly delayed—reaction* may include a rash with or without itching and hives, coughing, wheezing, painful joints, and swollen glands. Rarely, a severe (anaphylactic) reaction can occur with symptoms of nausea, facial swelling, difficulty breathing, abdominal pain, and shock. For more information, turn to page 79—SHOCK.

1. If the sting is from a honey bee, remove the stinger.

If the stinger is difficult to grasp, try to ease it out by gently scraping against the stinger with a fingernail, credit card, or table knife. Don't try to squeeze it with tweezers. If it is too deep to remove, call your doctor for instructions.

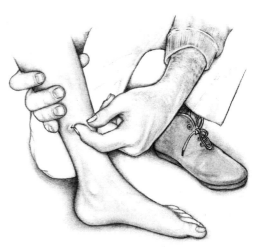

2. Wash the site with soap and lukewarm water.

   If calamine lotion, hydrocortisone cream or ointment, or baking soda and water (to make a paste) are available, apply some on the affected area to reduce discomfort.

   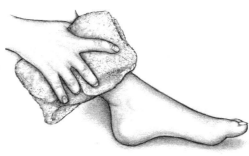

   Do not apply calamine lotion to your child's face or genitals.

3. Cover the site with a clean, cold compress or a clean, moist dressing to reduce swelling and discomfort.

4. Over the next 24 to 48 hours, observe the site for signs of infection (increasing redness, swelling, and pain).

   If the site becomes infected, call your doctor or take your child to an emergency room.

   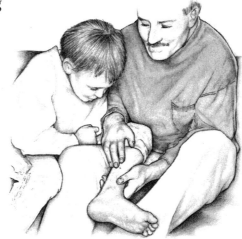

What to Check

- Observe your child's breathing and check the pulse. If needed, begin CPR:

  If your child is under 1 year old, see page 16, BREATHING/CARDIAC EMERGENCY, For Infant Under 1 Year.

  If your child is 1 to 8 years old, see page 20, BREATHING/CARDIAC EMERGENCY, For Child Age 1–8 Years.

  If your child is over 8 years old, see page 24, BREATHING/CARDIAC EMERGENCY, For Child Over 8 Years.

- If your child has a known history of serious reactions, check whether he is carrying an emergency medication such as an EpiPen or Twinject. Ask your child if your help is needed to administer the medication.

Bites & Stings

Snakebites

What You Need to Know

- Most snakebites are not poisonous. Most poisonous snakes—including rattlesnakes, copperheads, and water moccasins—have slit-like eyes. Coral snakes are a poisonous snake without slit-like eyes. The heads of poisonous snakes are triangular shaped and have a pit-like depression between the eyes and nostrils.

When to Get Professional Help

- If the bite is from a poisonous snake—or you are uncertain whether the snake is poisonous—call your local emergency number, or take your child to a hospital, immediately. Time is of the essence. If possible, call the hospital so antivenin can be ready when you arrive.

Signs & Symptoms

- One or two fang marks in the skin; burning, swelling, pain, or discoloration.
- *If venom enters the bloodstream*, nausea and vomiting may occur and progress to shock (clammy skin; rapid, shallow breathing; weak, rapid pulse). For more information, turn to page 79—SHOCK.

1. Keep your child calm, restrict her movement, and keep the affected area below heart level to reduce the flow of venom. Remove any jewelry in the area before swelling occurs.

2. Cleanse but do not flush the wound. Cover the bite with a clean, cool compress or a clean, moist dressing to reduce swelling and discomfort.

Consider applying a splint to help reduce discomfort. Turn to page ix—HOW TO MAKE A SPLINT.

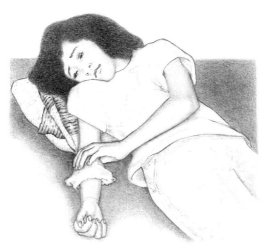

What to Check
- Observe your child's breathing and check the pulse. If needed, begin CPR:

  If your child is under 1 year old, see page 16, BREATHING/CARDIAC EMERGENCY, For Infant Under 1 Year.

  If your child is 1 to 8 years old, see page 20, BREATHING/CARDIAC EMERGENCY, For Child Age 1–8 Years.

  If your child is over 8 years old, see page 24, BREATHING/CARDIAC EMERGENCY, For Child Over 8 Years.

Don'ts
- Don't give your child anything by mouth.
- Don't apply ice to the bite.
- Don't apply a tourniquet, make incisions in the wound, or suction the venom; doing so may cause more harm than good.
- Don't try to capture the snake.

Bleeding

Cuts, Scrapes, Puncture Wounds, and Blisters

What You Need to Know

- Direct pressure will stop most bleeding. Minor cuts and scrapes usually stop bleeding on their own.
- Bleeding from the scalp is not always as serious as it seems; a small cut can appear to bleed profusely.
- Puncture wounds might not seem serious and often do not cause extensive bleeding; however, debris and germs can be carried through these wounds into tissues below the skin surface, resulting in infection. Puncture wounds on the foot are especially prone to infection.

What to Check

- Remember to check your child's ABC (airway, breathing, and circulation).
- If the bleeding cannot be controlled, observe your child for shock. If the child becomes dizzy or faint and/or develops pale, cool, clammy skin; rapid, shallow breathing; and a weak, rapid pulse, continue to treat the bleeding and turn to page 79—SHOCK.
- Check the status of your child's tetanus immunity.

1. Calm and reassure your child.

2. Apply direct, gentle pressure to the wound with a clean, dry cloth or bandage.

   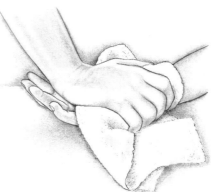

   Maintain firm but gentle pressure continuously for up to 20 to 30 minutes or until the bleeding subsides. If blood soaks through the cloth, don't remove it; you may loosen the clot. Place another cloth over the first one.

   Don't release pressure too often to check the wound, as this may also loosen or damage the clot. If blood continues to spurt after continuous pressure, seek medical attention.

3. If the wound is superficial, rinse it with clear water. Use a washcloth to clean the area around the wound with soap and warm water, then pat dry.

   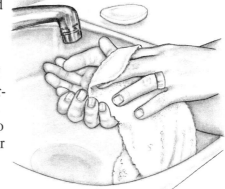

   Try to keep soap out of the wound, as it may irritate it. Use a tweezers cleaned with alcohol to remove visible debris or dirt in the wound.

   Don't wash a wound that is deep or bleeding profusely. If you are unsure about the seriousness of the wound, call your doctor.

A blister should be left intact unless it is very painful. It can be covered with a loose or porous bandage to keep it clean and protected. To break a painful blister, wash your hands with soap and water and swab the blister with rubbing alcohol. Sterilize a needle with rubbing alcohol. Puncture the blister at several spots along its edge; leave the overlying skin intact. Apply antibiotic ointment.

4. When the bleeding has subsided, even if the wound is still oozing, place a thin layer of antibiotic cream or ointment and place a clean dressing over the wound.

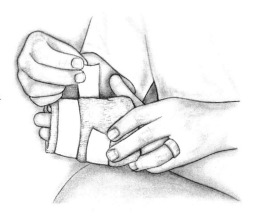

Bandage the dressing firmly, but not so tightly that the child's skin beyond the wound becomes pale and cool, which indicates that the circulation is being cut off.

5. Change the dressing whenever it becomes dirty or wet and at least once a day.

Watch for signs of infection including fever, redness, warmth, swelling, odor, or oozing. When the wound has healed enough to not become infected, leave it uncovered to speed healing.

When to Get Professional Help

- If the bleeding can't be controlled or is associated with a serious injury, call your local emergency number.
- If you think the wound might need stitches, or if embedded gravel or dirt cannot be removed easily with gentle cleaning, take your child to an emergency facility. Prompt treatment (within a few hours) is important to avoid secondary infection.
- Stitches may be needed to close cuts more than ¼ inch deep, cuts where fat or muscle is protruding, long or jagged cuts, cuts that are gaping open, cuts over joints, or cuts that may have damaged underlying tendons or nerves.

Don'ts

- Don't apply a tourniquet to control bleeding; doing so may cause more harm than good.

Breathing/Cardiac Emergency
For Infant Under 1 Year

What You Need to Know

- The procedures for CPR (cardiopulmonary resuscitation) described on page 19 are not a substitute for CPR training; they are performed most effectively and safely by those trained in CPR.
- In infants, most cardiac arrests are secondary to lack of oxygen such as occurs with respiratory failure, drowning, or choking.
- Rescue breathing is necessary for breathing/cardiac emergencies in infants. (See Step 5.) Administering only chest compressions does not work to resuscitate infants.
- If choking is the cause of breathing difficulty, follow the procedures on page 32—CHOKING, For Unconscious Infant Under 1 Year.

1. Rub or stroke your infant's back or tap her shoulder to determine whether she is conscious. Don't shake her to look for a response.

2. If she doesn't respond, turn her on her back onto a firm, flat surface in one motion, keeping her back in a straight line and firmly supporting her head and neck. Expose her chest.

   Remember to assess her ABC (airway, breathing, and circulation).

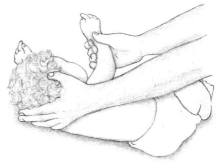

16

3. Lift your infant's chin gently with one hand while pushing down on the forehead with the other hand to tilt the head back. Be careful to not tilt the head back too far (which may block the airway).

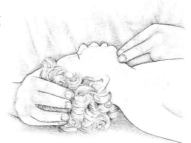

If you suspect a head, neck, or spinal injury, use the **chin lift maneuver**: *Do not tilt the head back*. Instead, gently lift the chin to pull the jaw forward and open the airway. Don't let her mouth close.

4. Place your ear close to your infant's mouth and watch for chest movement. For 5 to 10 seconds, look, listen, and feel for breathing on your cheek and ear.

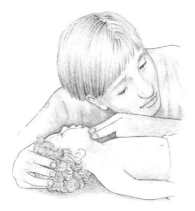

5. If she is not breathing, begin rescue breathing, as follows:

Maintain her head position and cover her mouth and nose tightly with your mouth. Give one slow, gentle breath, lasting 1 to 1½ seconds. Don't take a deep breath before giving rescue breathing; gently deliver just enough air to make your infant's chest rise.

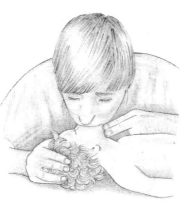

Don'ts

- Don't give chest compressions if there is a heartbeat; doing so may cause the heart to stop beating.
- If you suspect a head, neck, or spinal injury, *do not tilt back your child's head*. Use only the **chin lift maneuver**. (See Step 3.)
- Don't use an automated external defibrillator (AED) on a child younger than 1 year.

Continue to the next page

When to Get Professional Help

- If you are not alone, have one person call your local emergency number immediately while another person begins CPR.
- If you are alone, shout for help! If you are trained in CPR, administer CPR for about 2 minutes, then call your local emergency number.
- If you are alone and not trained in CPR, call your local emergency number immediately—emergency personnel will tell you what to do.

6. If you see her chest rise, give a second breath. If you don't see her chest rise, reposition her head, or redo the **chin lift maneuver** if you suspect a head, neck, or spinal injury. Give another breath. If her chest still doesn't rise, her airway is obstructed. Turn to page 32—CHOKING, For Unconscious Infant Under 1 Year.

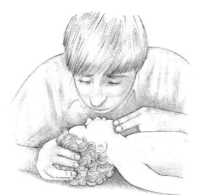

7. If you do see your infant's chest rise, place 2 fingers on the inside of her upper arm, just above the elbow. Squeeze gently to feel her pulse for 10 seconds. Keep in mind that that it is often difficult to quickly detect a pulse; if a pulse is not detected in 10 seconds, continue immediately to Step 9.

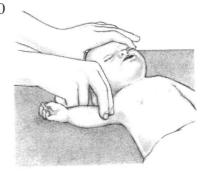

8. If she has a pulse, give 1 breath every 3 seconds. Check her pulse after every 20 breaths (each minute).

   After 1 minute, call your local emergency number. Resume giving breaths and checking the pulse.

9. If your infant has no pulse, begin chest compressions, as follows:

   Maintain her head position and place 2 fingers on the middle of her breastbone, just below the nipples. Within 3 seconds, quickly press your fingers down. The compression should be ⅓ to ½ the depth of the chest. The rate should be at least 100 compressions per minute (about 1½ to 2 compressions per second). Give the compressions in a smooth, rhythmic manner, keeping your fingers on her chest.

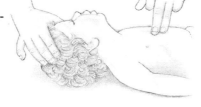

10. After 30 compressions, give 2 breaths. Repeat this sequence 5 times.

11. Recheck her pulse for 5 to 10 seconds.

12. Repeat Steps 10 and 11 until your infant's pulse resumes or help arrives. If her pulse resumes, go to Step 8.

Breathing/Cardiac Emergency

For Child Age 1–8 Years

What You Need to Know

- The procedures for CPR (cardiopulmonary resuscitation) described on page 23 are not a substitute for CPR training; they are performed most effectively and safely by those trained in CPR. If you do not feel adequately skilled in rescue breathing (see Step 5), it is acceptable to administer only chest compressions to resuscitate children older than 1 year.
- If choking is the cause of breathing difficulty, follow the procedures on page 38—CHOKING, For Unconscious Child Over 1 Year.

1. To determine consciousness, tap or shake your child gently and call his name or ask him, "Are you okay?"

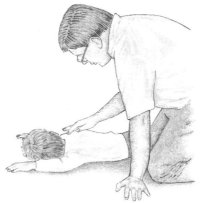

2. If he doesn't respond, turn him on his back onto a firm, flat surface in one motion, keeping his back in a straight line and firmly supporting his head and neck. Expose his chest.

    Remember to assess his ABC (airway, breathing, and circulation).

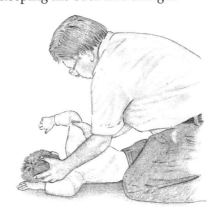

3. Lift your child's chin gently with one hand while pushing down on the forehead with the other hand to tilt the head back.

    If you suspect a head, neck, or spinal injury, use the **chin lift maneuver**: *Do not tilt the head back.* Instead, gently lift the chin to pull the jaw forward and open the airway. Don't let his mouth close.

4. Place your ear close to your child's mouth and watch for chest movement. For 5 to 10 seconds, look, listen, and feel for breathing on your cheek and ear.

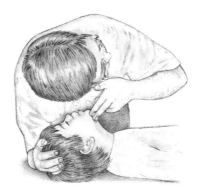

Don'ts

- Don't give chest compressions if there is a heartbeat; doing so may cause the heart to stop beating.
- If you suspect a head, neck, or spinal injury, *do not tilt back your child's head*. Use only the **chin lift maneuver**. (See Step 3.)

5. If he is not breathing, begin rescue breathing, as follows:

Maintain his head position, close his nostrils by pinching them with your thumb and index finger, and cover his mouth tightly with your mouth. Give 2 slow, gentle breaths, pausing after the first breath to inhale and exhaling just enough air to make his chest rise.

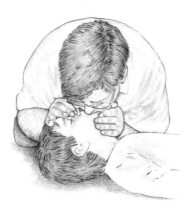

6. If you don't see his chest rise, reposition his head or redo the **chin lift maneuver** if you suspect a head, neck, or spinal injury. Give 2 more breaths.

If his chest still doesn't rise, his airway is obstructed. Turn to page 38—CHOKING, For Unconscious Child Over 1 Year.

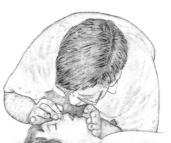

When to Get Professional Help

- If you are not alone, have one person call your local emergency number immediately and get an automated external defibrillator (AED) if available (preferably one with pediatric pads), while another person begins CPR.
- If you are alone, shout for help! If you are trained in CPR, administer CPR for about 1 minute, then call your local emergency number.
- If you are alone and not trained in CPR, call your local emergency number immediately—emergency personnel will tell you what to do.

7. If you do see your child's chest rise, place 2 fingers on his Adam's apple. Slide your fingers into the groove between the Adam's apple and the muscle on the side of his neck to feel his pulse for 10 seconds. Keep in mind that that it is often difficult to quickly detect a pulse; if a pulse is not detected in 10 seconds, continue immediately to Step 9.

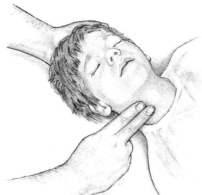

8. If he has a pulse, give 1 breath every 4 seconds. Check his pulse after every 15 breaths.

   After 1 minute, call your local emergency number. Resume giving breaths and checking the pulse.

9. If your child has no pulse, begin chest compressions, as follows:

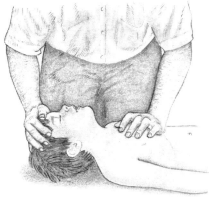

   Maintain his head position and place the heel of your hand on the breastbone, about level with his nipples. Lean your shoulders over your hand and within 4 seconds quickly press down. The compressions should be ⅓ to ½ the depth of the chest. The rate should be about 100 compressions per minute (about 1½ to 2 compressions per second). Give the compressions in a smooth, rhythmic manner, keeping your hand on his chest.

10. After 30 compressions, give 2 breaths. Repeat this sequence 5 times (about 2 minutes of resuscitation).

11. Recheck his pulse for 5 to 10 seconds.

    If your child's pulse hasn't resumed, apply an AED if available and follow the prompts. Administer one shock. Check for a pulse for no more than 10 seconds; if one isn't detected, administer a second shock.

12. Repeat Steps 10 and 11 until your child's pulse resumes or help arrives. If his pulse resumes, go to Step 8.

Continue to the next page

Breathing/Cardiac Emergency
For Child Over 8 Years

What You Need to Know

- The procedures for CPR (cardiopulmonary resuscitation) described on page 26 are not a substitute for CPR training; they are performed most effectively and safely by those trained in CPR. If you do not feel adequately skilled in rescue breathing (see Step 5), it is acceptable to administer only chest compressions to resuscitate children older than 1 year.
- If choking is the cause of breathing difficulty, follow the procedures on page 38—CHOKING, For Unconscious Child Over 1 Year.

1. To determine consciousness, tap or shake your child gently and call her name or ask her, "Are you okay?"

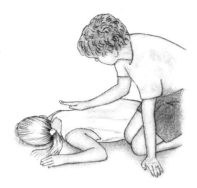

2. If she doesn't respond, turn her on her back in one motion onto a firm and flat surface, keeping her back in a straight line and firmly supporting her head and neck. Expose her chest.

   Remember to assess her ABC (airway, breathing, and circulation).

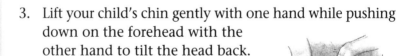

3. Lift your child's chin gently with one hand while pushing down on the forehead with the other hand to tilt the head back.

   If you suspect a head, neck, or spinal injury, use the **chin lift maneuver**: *Do not tilt the head back.* Instead, gently lift the chin to pull the jaw forward and open the airway. Don't let her mouth close.

4. Place your ear close to your child's mouth and watch for chest movement. For 5 to 10 seconds, look, listen, and feel for breathing.

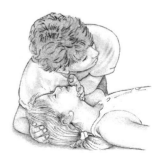

24

5. If she is not breathing, begin rescue breathing, as follows:

Maintain her head position, close her nostrils by pinching them with your thumb and index finger, and cover her mouth tightly with your mouth. Give 2 slow, full breaths, pausing after the first breath to inhale deeply.

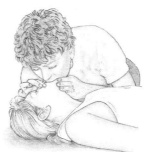

Don'ts
- Don't give chest compressions if there is a heartbeat; doing so may cause the heart to stop beating.
- If you suspect a head, neck, or spinal injury, *do not tilt back your child's head*. Use only the **chin lift maneuver**. (See Step 3.)

6. If you don't see her chest rise, reposition her head or redo the **chin lift maneuver** if you suspect a head, neck, or spinal injury. Give 2 more breaths.

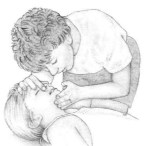

If her chest still doesn't rise, her airway is obstructed. Turn to page 38—CHOKING, For Unconscious Child Over 1 Year.

7. If you do see your child's chest rise, place 2 fingers on her Adam's apple. Slide your fingers into the groove between the Adam's apple and the muscle on the side of her neck to feel her pulse for 10 seconds. Keep in mind that that it is often difficult to quickly detect a pulse; if a pulse is not detected in 10 seconds, continue immediately to Step 9.

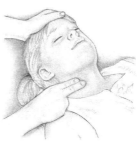

8. If she has a pulse, give 1 breath every 5 seconds. Check her pulse after every 12 breaths.

After 1 minute, call your local emergency number. Resume giving breaths and checking the pulse.

Continue to the next page

When to Get Professional Help

- If you are not alone, have one person call your local emergency number immediately and get an automated external defibrillator (AED) if available (preferably one with pediatric pads), while another person begins CPR.
- If you are alone, shout for help! If you are trained in CPR, administer CPR for about 2 minutes, then call your local emergency number.
- If you are alone and not trained in CPR, call your local emergency number immediately—emergency personnel will tell you what to do.

9. If your child has no pulse, begin chest compressions, as follows:

   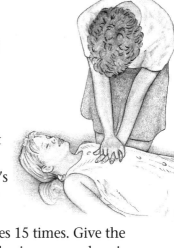

   Maintain her head position and place the heel of your hand 2 finger-widths above the lowest notch of her breastbone. Place the heel of your other hand directly over the heel of the first hand. Interlock your fingers; don't let them touch your child's chest. Lean your shoulders over your hands, and within 10 seconds quickly press down 2 inches 15 times. Give the compressions in a smooth, rhythmic manner, keeping your hands on her chest.

10. Give your child 2 full breaths, followed by 30 chest compressions. Repeat this sequence 5 times.

11. Recheck her pulse for 5 to 10 seconds.

    If an AED is available, use it as instructed .

12. Repeat Steps 10 and 11 until your child's pulse resumes or help arrives. If her pulse resumes, go to Step 8.

Burns

Signs & Symptoms
- *First-degree* burns affect the outer layer of the skin, causing pain, redness, and swelling.
- *Second-degree* burns affect both the outer and underlying layer of the skin, causing pain, redness and blotchiness, swelling, and blistering. Typically, the perimeter of the burn measures more than three inches.
- *Third-degree* burns extend into deeper tissues, may cause brown or blackened skin, and may be painless. They are likely to cause permanent tissue damage.

1. If your child has a *chemical burn*, brush away any dry chemical, immediately remove all burned clothing and jewelry, and rinse the burned area in cool water under a tap, hose, or shower for 20 minutes.

   Pat dry. Go to Step 4.

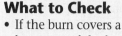

What to Check
- If the burn covers a large part of the body, observe your child for shock. Turn to page 79—SHOCK if the child becomes dizzy or faint and/or develops pale, cool, clammy skin; rapid, shallow breathing; and a weak, rapid pulse.
- Find out if your child's tetanus immunity is up to date.

Don'ts
- Don't remove dead skin or break blisters.
- Don't apply ice, butter, ointments, medications, fluffy cotton dressings, or adhesive bandages to a burn.

Continue to the next page

- If you have any concerns about a burn, call your local emergency number.
- For any burn from a fire, or any chemical or electrical burn, or if you are uncertain about the burn's severity, call your doctor or go to an emergency facility.
- If your child has been burned on the face, scalp, hands, feet, joints or genitals, go to an emergency facility.

2. If your child is *on fire*, either (a) douse her with water if it is available; (b) wrap her in thick, nonsynthetic material such as a wool or cotton coat, rug, or blanket to smother the flames; or (c) lay her flat and roll her on the ground.

   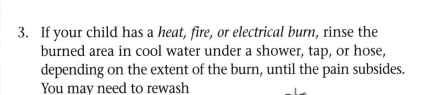

   If your clothes catch fire, STOP, DROP, AND ROLL. When the fire is out, go to Step 3.

3. If your child has a *heat, fire, or electrical burn*, rinse the burned area in cool water under a shower, tap, or hose, depending on the extent of the burn, until the pain subsides. You may need to rewash areas if pain recurs.

   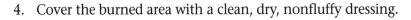

   Cover burned areas that cannot be immersed, such as the face, with wet cloths. Pat dry.

4. Cover the burned area with a clean, dry, nonfluffy dressing.

   If the burn is on your child's hands or feet, keep her fingers or toes apart by placing cloth or gauze between them; then loosely wrap the hand or foot in a clean dressing.

   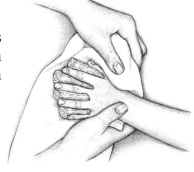

5. If the burn is minor, over the next 24 to 48 hours observe the area for signs of infection (increasing redness, swelling, and pain).

    If the burn looks infected, call your doctor or take your child to an emergency facility.

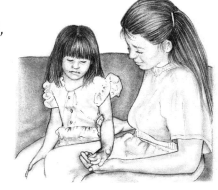

6. If the burn is extensive and your child is not vomiting, give her liquids to help replace lost fluids.

    Give pain-relieving medication (acetaminophen or ibuprofen) as necessary. Follow the dosage and age recommendations on the package label.

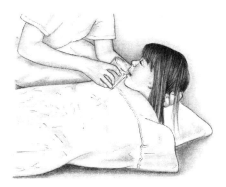

Choking

For Conscious Infant Under 1 Year

What You Need to Know

- Choking occurs when something blocks the airway. It can be food or (especially with young children) small objects. Choking can seem very frightening, but quick action can help restore breathing.

When to Get Professional Help

- If you are not alone, have one person call your local emergency number while another person follows the first-aid steps below.
- If you are alone and can do so quickly, call your local emergency number. Then follow these first-aid steps.
- Even if you successfully dislodge the obstruction and your infant seems fine, call your doctor for further instructions.

Signs & Symptoms

- Inability to breathe, cry, or make sounds; high-pitched noises; silent, ineffective coughs; face becomes blue; loss of consciousness.

1. Assume a seated position and lay your infant face down along your forearm with his chest in your hand and his jaw between your thumb and index finger. Use your thigh or lap for support. Keep his head lower than his body.

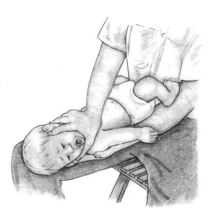

2. Give 5 quick, forceful blows, one a second, between his shoulder blades with the heel of your other hand.

   Gravity and the force of the back blows should release the blocking object.

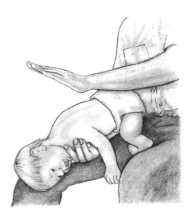

3. While supporting the head, turn your infant over so he is face up on your other arm. Use your thigh or lap for support. Keep his head lower than his body.

4. Place 2 or 3 fingers on the center of his breastbone. Avoid the tip of the breastbone.

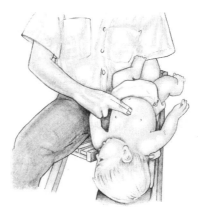

5. Quickly thrust your fingers down ½ to 1 inch 5 times.

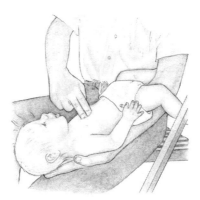

6. If the object does not come out, turn your infant over so he is face down on your other arm and give another 5 back blows.

Continue alternating 5 back blows with 5 chest thrusts until the object is dislodged, help arrives, or your infant loses consciousness.

If your infant loses consciousness, turn to the next page—CHOKING, For Unconscious Infant Under 1 Year.

Don'ts

- Don't interfere with your infant if he can still cough, breathe, talk, or cry.
- Don't try to dislodge and remove the object if you cannot see it. (If you can see the object, try to dislodge and remove it with your hooked index finger.)
- Don't initiate these first-aid steps until you are certain your infant is actually choking. If he can't cough or cry, sputter, or move air, then follow these first-aid steps.

Choking

For Unconscious Infant Under 1 Year

What to Check

- Rub your infant's back or tap his shoulder to determine whether he is conscious. If he doesn't respond, then follow these first-aid steps.

Don'ts

- Don't try to dislodge and remove the object if you cannot see it.
- Never shake an infant to determine whether he is conscious.

1. Firmly supporting your infant's head and neck with one hand, place him on his back in one motion onto a hard surface, keeping his back in a straight line. Expose his chest.

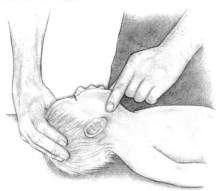

2. Put your thumb in your infant's mouth and grasp the lower teeth or gums, lifting the jaw upward. *If the object is visible and loose*, remove it. Be careful not to push the object deeper into the airway—this can happen easily in infants and young children.

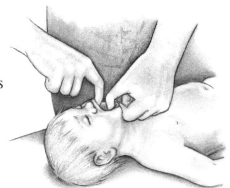

3. Look, listen, and feel for breathing.

Lift your infant's chin while tilting his head back to move his tongue away from his windpipe. Don't let his mouth close. Place your ear close to his mouth and watch for chest movement. For 5 seconds, look, listen, and feel for breathing.

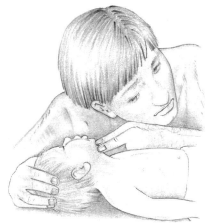

4. If your infant is not breathing, begin rescue breathing, as follows:

   Maintain his head position and cover his mouth and nose tightly with your mouth. Give 2 slow, gentle breaths, each lasting 1 to 1½ seconds with a pause in between in which you take a breath.

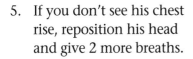

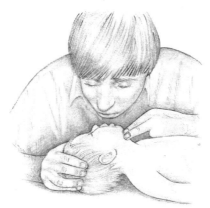

5. If you don't see his chest rise, reposition his head and give 2 more breaths.

When to Get Professional Help

- If you are not alone, have one person call your local emergency number while another person follows these first-aid steps.
- If you are alone, shout for help! If you can do so quickly, call your local emergency number. Then follow these first-aid steps.
- Even if you successfully dislodge the obstruction and your infant seems fine, call your doctor for further instructions.

Continue to the next page

6. If your infant's chest still doesn't rise, begin back blows.

   Lay him face down along your forearm with his chest in your hand and his jaw between your thumb and index finger. Use your thigh or lap for support. Keep his head lower than his body.

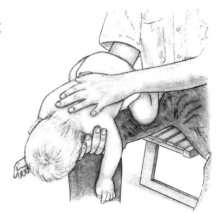

7. Give 5 quick, forceful blows between his shoulder blades with the heel of your other hand.

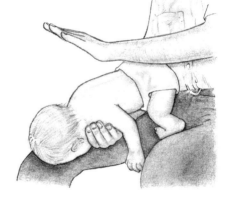

8. Turn your infant over so he is face up on your other arm. Use your thigh or lap for support. Keep his head lower than his body.

9. Place 2 fingers on the lower half of his breastbone, one finger's breadth below his nipples.

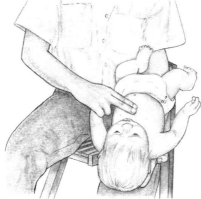

10. Quickly thrust your fingers down 1 inch 5 times at the rate of one a second.

11. Open your infant's mouth with your thumb and index finger, placing your thumb over his tongue. *If the object is visible and loose,* remove it. Observe his breathing.

    If your infant stops breathing, begin CPR (see page 16—BREATHING/CARDIAC EMERGENCY, For Infant Under 1 Year).

12. If the object is not dislodged, give 2 breaths, 5 back blows, 5 chest thrusts, and then check for the object. Repeat this sequence until the object is dislodged or help arrives.

Choking

For Conscious Child Over 1 Year

When to Get Professional Help

- If you are not alone, have one person call your local emergency number while another person follows these first-aid steps.
- If you are alone and can do so quickly, call your local emergency number. Then follow these first-aid steps.
- Even if you successfully dislodge the obstruction and your child seems fine, call your doctor for further instructions.

Signs & Symptoms

- Inability to breathe, talk, or cry; high-pitched noises; ineffective coughs; face becomes blue.

1. Stand behind your child and wrap your arms around her waist. Tip her forward slightly.

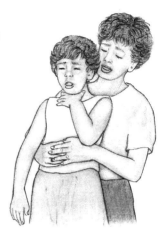

2. Make a fist with one of your hands. Grasp the fist with your other hand. Place the thumb-side of your fist in the middle of your child's abdomen, just above the navel and well below the tip of her breastbone and ribs.

3. Keep your elbows out and press your fist into your child's abdomen inward and upward with a series of 5 quick, distinct thrusts as if trying to lift the child up. Do not touch the breastbone or rib cage. This is also known as the Heimlich maneuver.

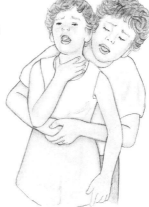

Don'ts

- Don't interfere with your child if she can still cough, breathe, talk, or cry.
- Don't try to dislodge and remove the object if you cannot see it.
- Don't initiate these first-aid steps until you are certain your child is actually choking. Encourage coughing to clear the airway. If she can't cough or her cough is very weak, then follow these first-aid steps.

4. Continue these abdominal thrusts until the object is dislodged, help arrives, or your child loses consciousness.

If your child loses consciousness, turn to the next page—CHOKING, For Unconscious Child Over 1 Year.

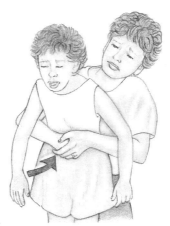

Choking
For Unconscious Child Over 1 Year

What to Check

- Tap or shake your child gently and call her name to determine whether she is conscious. If she doesn't respond, then follow these first-aid steps.

Don'ts

- Don't try to dislodge and remove the object if you cannot see it.

1. Firmly supporting your child's head and neck, place her on her back onto a firm, flat surface in one motion, keeping her back in a straight line. Expose her chest.

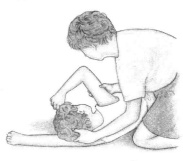

2. Open your child's mouth with your thumb and index finger, placing your thumb over her tongue. *If the object is visible and loose*, remove it. Be careful not to push the object deeper into the airway—this can happen easily in young children.

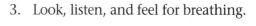

3. Look, listen, and feel for breathing.

   Lift your child's chin while tilting her head back to move her tongue away from her windpipe. Don't let her mouth close. Place your ear close to her mouth and watch for chest movement. For 5 seconds, look, listen, and feel for breathing.

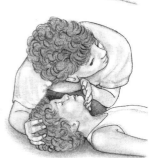

4. If your child is not breathing, begin rescue breathing, as follows:

   Maintain her head position, close her nostrils by pinching them with your thumb and index finger, and cover her mouth tightly with your mouth. Give 2 slow breaths, with a pause in between in which you take a breath.

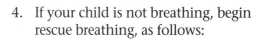
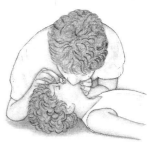

5. If you don't see her chest rise, reposition her head and give 2 more breaths.

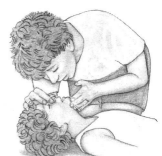

6. If your child's chest still doesn't rise, begin abdominal thrusts, as follows:

   Kneel at her feet or astride her thighs. Place the heel of your hand in the middle of her abdomen just above her navel but well below the tip of her breastbone and rib cage. Place your other hand on top of the first hand.

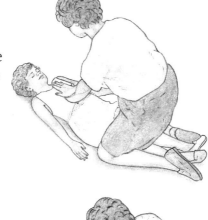

When to Get Professional Help
- If you are not alone, have one person call your local emergency number while another person follows these first-aid steps.
- If you are alone, shout for help! If you can do so quickly, call your local emergency number. Then follow these first-aid steps.
- Even if you successfully dislodge the obstruction and your child seems fine, call your doctor for further instructions.

7. Press into your child's abdomen with a series of 5 quick, continuous upward thrusts.

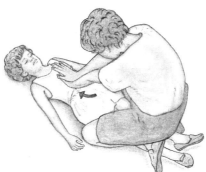

8. Open your child's mouth with your thumb and index finger. *If the object is visible and loose,* remove it with a hooked index finger. Observe her breathing.

   If your child stops breathing, begin CPR:

   If your child is 1 to 8 years old, see page 20—BREATHING/ CARDIAC EMERGENCY, For Child Age 1–8 Years.

   If your child is over 8 years old, see page 24—BREATHING/ CARDIAC EMERGENCY, For Child Over 8 Years.

9. If the object is not dislodged, give 2 breaths, 5 abdominal thrusts, and then check for the object. Repeat this sequence until the object is dislodged or help arrives.

Cold Emergencies
Frostbite

What You Need to Know

- Frostbite occurs when the skin and underlying tissues freeze.
- Frostbite most frequently affects exposed areas, such as the fingers, toes, ears, nose, and cheeks.
- Frostbite occurs in three stages: frostnip, superficial frostbite, and severe frostbite.

What to Check

- Your child may also have hypothermia. If the child is shivering uncontrollably, turn immediately to page 42—COLD EMERGENCIES, Hypothermia.

Signs & Symptoms

- Numbness, itchiness, pain and burning, hard or waxy skin, yellowish white or grayish yellow color to skin, blisters.
- Clumsiness can occur due to stiff muscles and joints.
- As the skin thaws, it becomes red and painful.

1. Take your child indoors as soon as possible, remove wet clothing from the affected area, and remove any rings from frostbitten hands.

   If you cannot get indoors, try to protect the frostbitten skin from further exposure. Tuck frostbitten hands in armpits. Cover other exposed areas with dry, gloved hands, if possible.

2. Immerse affected areas in warm (not hot) water (104°F to 107.6°F or 40°C to 42°C)—or apply warm cloths or blankets to affected ears, nose, or cheeks—for 20 to 30 minutes.

   Add water as needed to maintain water temperature. Your child will probably complain of intense pain as thawing progresses. After thawing, pat affected parts dry.
   - If feeling and color return, no further treatment is needed.
   - If feeling and color do not return, or if there are blisters, call your doctor and continue with Steps 3 through 5.

3. Wrap affected hands or feet loosely in a clean dressing.

Keep fingers or toes apart by placing cloth or gauze between them before wrapping hands or feet. Be careful not to break blisters by rubbing.

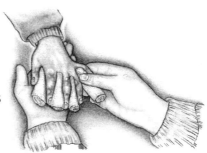

4. Elevate affected hands or feet.

Have your child try to move the affected parts to increase circulation. Don't let him walk if his feet are affected.

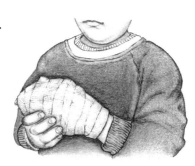

5. If the frostbite is extensive, give your child warm liquids to replace lost fluids.

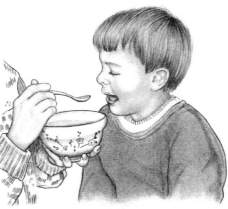

When to Get Professional Help

- Call your doctor or take your child to an emergency facility if you think that the cold exposure was prolonged, or if your child has a fever or experiences dizziness, achiness, increased pain, swelling, redness, or discharge in the frostbitten areas.

Don'ts

- Don't treat affected parts with hot water or a dry heat source such as a hair dryer, space heater, fireplace, stove, or heating pad. This may cause burns.
- Don't rub or massage affected parts or break blisters.
- Don't thaw affected parts if you are outdoors and refreezing could occur.
- Don't rub snow on affected skin.
- Don't let your child walk on frostbitten toes or feet; this may damage tissue.

Cold Emergencies
Hypothermia

What You Need to Know

- Hypothermia occurs when more heat is lost from the body than it can regenerate.
- Symptoms usually develop slowly.
- Infants, young children, and those with lean body types are at increased risk to develop hypothermia.
- Bodies lose heat much faster in cold water or through wet clothing than when dry.
- Exposure to a high wind-chill factor, high humidity, or cool, damp environments can increase the risk of hypothermia.

What to Check

- Observe your child for shock. If she becomes dizzy or faint and/or develops pale, cool, clammy skin; rapid, shallow breathing; and a weak, rapid pulse, turn to page 79—SHOCK.

Signs & Symptoms

- Uncontrollable shivering, cool and pale skin, weakness, lethargy, apathy, memory loss, drowsiness, confusion, slurred speech, slowing of breathing, or shock.
- Infants may develop bright red, cold skin.
- Very low body temperature—less than 95°F (35°C).

1. Bring your child into a warm room (if in the woods, start a fire and create shelter from the wind and protect her body from the cold ground), remove any wet clothing, and keep her awake. Cover her head.

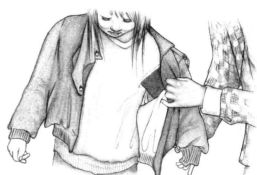

2. Apply warm compresses to the center of her body (the head, neck, chest wall, and groin). Don't try to warm the arms and legs as this may send cold blood to the central organs (heart, brain, and lungs).

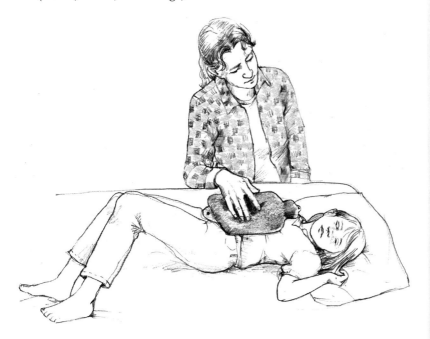

3. If your child is conscious and not vomiting, give her warm liquids.

When to Get Professional Help

- If you observe the signs and symptoms listed on page 42, if your child's temperature is less than 95°F (35°C), or if you think that cold exposure was prolonged, call your local emergency number.

Don'ts

- Don't massage or rub your child; handle her gently.
- Don't apply direct heat to her body.

Convulsion/Seizure

What You Need to Know

- Remain calm; most convulsions stop within 15 minutes, usually within 1 minute.
- Many childhood convulsions that occur between 6 months and 5 years of age are caused by fever (usually within the first few hours and when there is a rapid increase in temperature) and are not serious. Often there will be a family history of seizures occurring with fevers. Seizures that are not prolonged (over 30 to 45 minutes) do not cause brain damage.
- Some illnesses are more likely to present with seizures as a symptom, including pneumonia, meningitis, shigella infections, diarrhea, and roseola.
- If professional help is required, your child may undergo tests to evaluate the problem, including blood tests, urine tests, X-rays, and a spinal tap.

Signs & Symptoms

- Uncontrollable body movements, jerking, twitching, eyes rolled back, foaming at the mouth, clenched teeth, biting the cheek or tongue, staring, loss of bowel and bladder control, loss of consciousness.
- After a seizure, the child may be sleepy or experience memory loss, headache, or confusion.

1. If necessary, move your child to a safe place where he cannot be injured.

   If possible, lay him face up on the floor.

   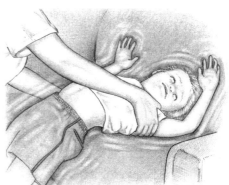

2. Stay with your child unless you need to obtain medical help.

   Loosen his clothing at the neck and the waist.

   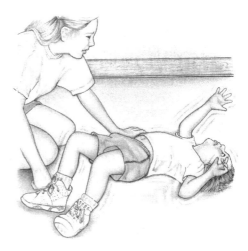

3. Place your child on his side if he vomits to prevent him from inhaling vomit or mucus into his lungs.

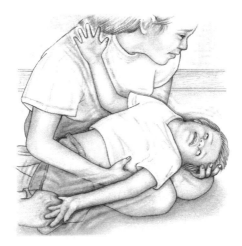

4. If the convulsion has stopped and your child feels feverish, turn to page 64—FEVER.

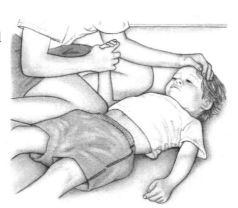

When to Get Professional Help

- If the convulsion lasts more than 5 minutes or your child is having repeated convulsions or trouble breathing, call your local emergency number.
- If the convulsion is your child's first, call your doctor.

Don'ts

- Don't restrain your child, try to force his mouth open, place your fingers in his mouth, and/or try to grasp his tongue.

Croup

What You Need to Know

- Croup is an infection, usually viral, that settles in the area of the voice box and windpipe. The infection causes inflammation and swelling, thus narrowing the windpipe.
- The symptoms of croup can come on gradually or suddenly, often waking infants and children in the middle of the night.
- Croup is most common between 6 months and 3 years of age, and occurs most frequently between the months of October and March in North America.

Don'ts

- Don't try to open your child's airway with your finger.
- Don't try to make your child vomit to clear the airway.

Signs & Symptoms

- "Barky" cough that sounds similar to the barking of a seal or dog; making a harsh, raspy, whooping sound when inhaling (stridor); drooling; loss of appetite; disinterest in drinking fluids; too tired to cough.

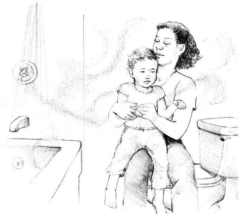

1. Take your child into the bathroom, close the door, and turn on the shower to the hottest setting, to let the bathroom steam up. Sit in the room with him for 15 to 20 minutes. The warm, moist air should help him breathe easier.

   Alternatively, you can expose him to cold, moist air by sitting with him outdoors if the conditions are appropriate. Cover him as needed to keep him from getting chilled.

   If the moist air exposure does not help his breathing, call your doctor. If at any point he becomes blue or struggles to breathe, call your local emergency number.

2. For the remainder of the night and for the next few nights, use a cold-water vaporizer or humidifier in the room where your child sleeps.

   Medication may be prescribed, usually a form of a steroid, to help decrease the swelling and inflammation. If so, give it to your child as directed.

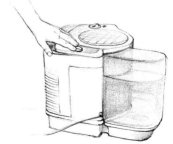

Dental Emergencies
Dislodged or Broken Permanent Tooth

Don'ts
- Don't rub or scrape the tooth to remove debris.
- Don't try to replant a baby tooth.

1. Handle the tooth by the top or crown, not by the roots.

    Gently rinse the tooth in a bowl of tap water. Don't hold it under running water.

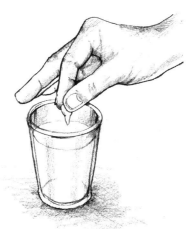

2. Try to replace the tooth in the socket immediately. If it doesn't go all the way in, have your child bite down slowly on a gauze and hold it in place until your child's dentist can see her.

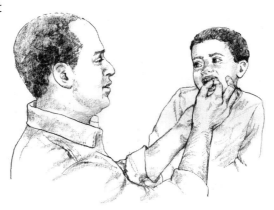

Continue to the next page

3. If you can't place the tooth in the socket, immediately place it in milk or a mild salt water solution by mixing ¼ teaspoon salt in 1 quart of water. Or place the tooth in a commercial container such as Save-A-Tooth (http://saveatooth.com). If the tooth is broken, save the broken part.

    Have you child rinse her mouth with warm water and apply cold compresses or cold packs.

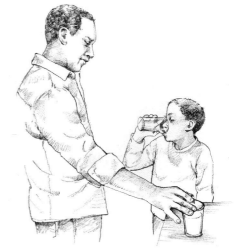

4. If there is a cut or bite on the tongue, lip, or cheek lining, clean the area with a clean cloth and apply cold compresses or cold packs as able.

5. Schedule an appointment with your child's dentist for as soon as possible.

Dental Emergencies
Toothache

1. Rinse your child's mouth with warm water.

   Use dental floss to remove any particles of food that may be present.

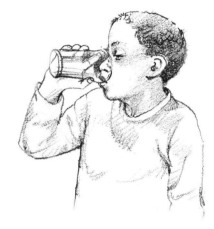

2. Apply a cold compress or cold pack to the affected area of the face.

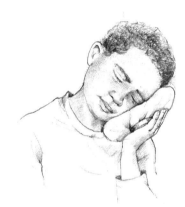

For additional pain relief, give your child acetaminophen or ibuprofen. Follow the dosage and age recommendations on the package label.

If available, apply an antiseptic medicine containing benzocaine to the affected area.

What You Need to Know

- The primary cause of a toothache is decay. Bacteria form a sticky plague that contains acids that can eat through the hard, white coating (enamel) of the tooth, causing a cavity. Very cold or hot liquids or sweets may precipitate the pain.

Don'ts

- Don't apply an aspirin or other pain medicine on the aching tooth.

When to Get Professional Help

- If fever, persisting pain, difficulty breathing, or trouble swallowing occurs, contact your child's dentist.

Drowning

Ice Rescue

When to Get Professional Help

- If possible, call your local emergency number immediately.
- After an ice rescue, if your child is unconscious, if he has been submerged for any period of time, if he is hypothermic (see page 42—COLD EMERGENCIES, Hypothermia), or if you have any concerns, call your local emergency number; otherwise, call your doctor.

Don'ts

- Don't go out on the ice to rescue a child you can reach with your arm or an extended object.
- Don't let a drowning child grab you; he might pull you under.

1. Have your child extend his arms flat on the ice and kick to keep afloat.

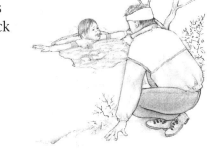

2. Kneel or lie down near the edge of the ice, brace yourself firmly, and reach for your child with your arm or an extended object such as a stick, a rope, or clothing.

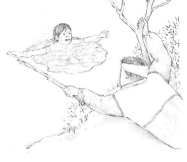

   If you must move onto the ice, lie flat and edge out slowly until the extended object is within the child's reach.

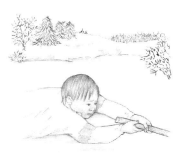

3. Have your child lie flat while you pull him to safety; don't let him get up and walk off the ice.

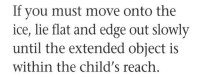

4. If you can't pull your child out with an extended object and other people are available, form a human chain to pull him out. Have everyone slide out on the ice lying flat and spread-eagled, grasping the ankles of the person in front.

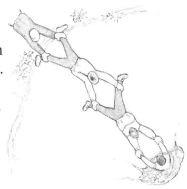

5. Observe your child's breathing, check the pulse, and give CPR if needed.

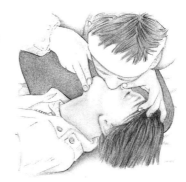

6. Expel fluids or objects by sweeping your finger along the inside of your child's mouth. If he vomits, turn his head to the side and remove the vomit from his mouth.

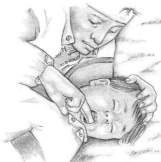

7. If your child is breathing, take him to a warm place, remove any wet clothing, wrap him in blankets, and call for professional help.

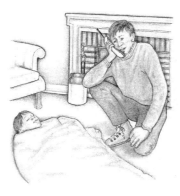

8. If your child is shivering uncontrollably, call your local emergency number and treat him for possible hypothermia.

Turn to page 42—COLD EMERGENCIES, Hypothermia.

What You Need to Know

- With ice rescue, time is of the essence. Submersion in ice water can rapidly lead to hypothermia.
- Give CPR if needed, even to a child who has been submerged for an extended period. Continue CPR until help arrives or your child begins to breathe on his own.

If your child is under 1 year old, see page 16, BREATHING/CARDIAC EMERGENCY, For Infant Under 1 Year.

If your child is 1 to 8 years old, see page 20, BREATHING/CARDIAC EMERGENCY, For Child Age 1–8 Years.

If your child is over 8 years old, see page 24, BREATHING/CARDIAC EMERGENCY, For Child Over 8 Years.

Drowning

Water Rescue

When to Get Professional Help

- If possible, check the area to alert a lifeguard and call your local emergency number immediately.
- After a water rescue, if your child is unconscious, if she has been submerged for any period of time, or if you have any concerns, call your local emergency number; otherwise, call your doctor.

Don'ts

- Don't enter the water to rescue a child who can be reached with your arm, a boat, an extended object, or a throwable object. Dangerous currents or riptides may also endanger you.
- Don't let a drowning child grab you; she might pull you under.

Signs & Symptoms

- Flailing, yelling for help, coughing, going under the water and struggling to surface, appearing unconscious, floating face down.

1. If your child is within reach, kneel or lie down near the edge of the water, brace yourself firmly, and reach for her with your arm or an extended object such as a pole, oar, or towel.

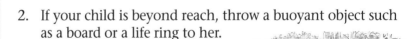

2. If your child is beyond reach, throw a buoyant object such as a board or a life ring to her.

   If possible, throw an object with a line attached so you can pull her in; try to throw the object past her and then pull it within her reach. If the object has no line, tell her to grab the object and kick to safety.

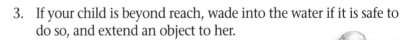

3. If your child is beyond reach, wade into the water if it is safe to do so, and extend an object to her.

   Either pull her to safety or, if the object is buoyant, let go of it and tell her to kick to safety. Be sure to keep the object between you and the child—don't let her grab you.

4. If you must swim to your child, keep your eye on the spot where you last saw her and bring an object for her to hold on to—don't let her grab you.

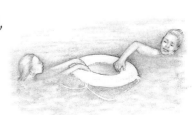

5. If your child is not breathing, begin mouth-to-mouth resuscitation—while still in the water if possible—and head for land. Once on land, check the pulse and give CPR if needed.

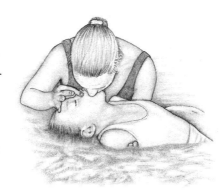

6. Expel fluids or objects by sweeping your finger along the inside of your child's mouth. If she vomits, turn her head to the side and remove the vomit from her mouth.

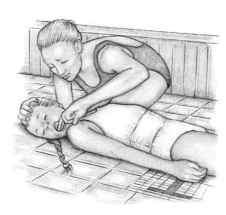

7. If your child is breathing, remove any wet clothing, wrap her in blankets, and call for professional help.

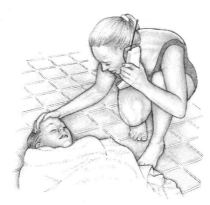

What You Need to Know

- A child who is drowning often cannot call out for help.
- Give CPR if needed, even to a child who has been submerged for an extended period, especially in cold water. Continue CPR until help arrives or your child begins to breathe on her own.

If your child is under 1 year old, see page 16, BREATHING/CARDIAC EMERGENCY, For Infant Under 1 Year.

If your child is 1 to 8 years old, see page 20, BREATHING/CARDIAC EMERGENCY, For Child Age 1–8 Years.

If your child is over 8 years old, see page 24, BREATHING/CARDIAC EMERGENCY, For Child Over 8 Years.

Earache

What You Need to Know

- Ear infections are very common in infancy and childhood and are often associated with colds. Trauma from scratching or inserting objects into the ear (for instance, for cleaning) can also cause infection.
- There are different types of ear infections and different causes. Types include outer ear infections (also called "swimmer's ear"), middle ear infections, and inner ear infections.
- Some middle ear infections cause drainage into the outer ear canal through a hole in the eardrum.

Signs & Symptoms

- Pain, irritability, prolonged or excessive crying, fever, dizziness, ringing in ear, discharge, hearing loss.

1. Give your child pain-relieving tablets or liquid (acetaminophen or ibuprofen).

   Follow the dosage and age guidelines recommended on the package label.

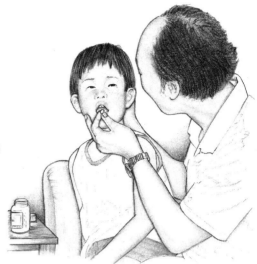

2. If previously prescribed, give your child eardrops for pain.

   Warm the bottle in your hand and lay the child on his back with his head turned to the side. Pull his ear up and out, and insert 3 or 4 drops in the ear canal. Place a small piece of cotton in his ear if tolerated. Keep him lying down with his head turned to the side for a few minutes to allow drops to come in contact with the eardrum.

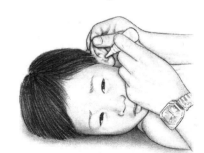

3. Apply a heating pad, warm washcloth, or hot-water bottle to the ear to reduce discomfort.

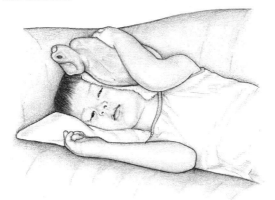

When to Get Professional Help

- If your child has an earache, call your doctor. Most ear infections, even mild ones, require treatment.

4. If your child is uncomfortable lying down, let him rest in an upright position (which reduces pressure in the middle ear and may help alleviate pain).

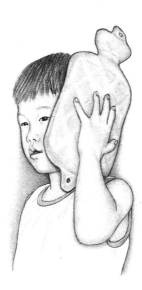

Electrical Injuries

Burns & Shock

What You Need to Know

- Causes of electrical injuries include exposure to household or appliance wiring or severed electrical cords, sticking foreign objects into outlets, and arcs from power lines.
- An electrical shock may be brief and harmless, or it may be life threatening.
- On the surface, an electrical injury may appear minor or not show at all, but it may extend deep into the interior and affect tissues and organs.

Don'ts

- Don't touch your child until you check that she is not still in contact with electrical current. Don't get anywhere near high-voltage wires until the power is turned off.
- Don't move your child unless she is in immediate danger.
- If burns are present, don't remove dead skin or break blisters.
- Don't apply ice, butter, ointments, medications, fluffy cotton dressings, or adhesive bandages to a burn.

Signs & Symptoms

- Skin burns, irregular heart rhythm, respiratory failure, muscle pain and contractions, seizures, numbness and tingling, loss of consciousness, weakness, and fractures.

1. Unplug the cord or turn off the power at the circuit or breaker box.

   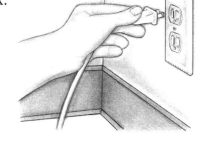

   Your child might not be able to let go of the point of contact if her muscles have contracted strongly in response to the electricity.

2. If the current can't be turned off, use a dry, nonconducting object made of cardboard, plastic, or wood (such as a broom, chair, rug, or rubber doormat) to move the source of the current away from your child.

   Don't use a wet or metal object. If possible, stand on something dry and nonconducting, such as a mat or folded newspapers.

   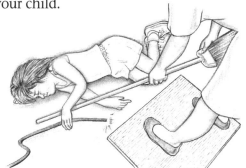

3. Check your child's ABC (airway, breathing, and circulation). Position her on her back and elevate her feet, to help prevent shock.

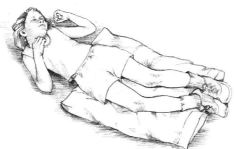

4. If there is a skin burn, cover the burned area with a clean, dry, nonfluffy dressing. Don't use a blanket or towel with loose fibers that might stick to the burn.

If the burn is on your child's hand or foot, keep her fingers or toes apart by placing cloth or gauze between them; then loosely wrap the hand or foot in a clean dressing.

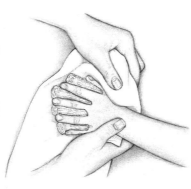

When to Get Professional Help
- If your child is unconscious, is in significant pain, has difficulty breathing, or has extensive electrical burns, call your local emergency number.
- If your child has come into contact with electricity, have your doctor check her for internal injuries.

What to Check
- Observe your child for signs of shock. If she becomes dizzy or faint and/or develops pale, cool, clammy skin; rapid, shallow breathing; and a weak, rapid pulse, turn to page 79—SHOCK.
- Observe your child's breathing and check the pulse. If needed, begin CPR:

If your child is under 1 year old, see page 16, BREATHING/CARDIAC EMERGENCY, For Infant Under 1 Year.

If your child is 1 to 8 years old, see page 20, BREATHING/CARDIAC EMERGENCY, For Child Age 1–8 Years.

If your child is over 8 years old, see page 24, BREATHING/CARDIAC EMERGENCY, For Child Over 8 Years.

Eye Emergencies
Chemical Injury

- Prompt flushing of the eye is important.

When to Get Professional Help

- If any chemicals get in your child's eye, take your child to an emergency facility and bring the chemical container or name of the chemical with you. Have your child wear sunglasses; his eyes may be sensitive.

Don'ts

- Don't rub the eye, as this may cause more damage.
- Don't use eyedrops unless instructed to do so.

1. Turn your child's head so the injured eye is down and to the side. Holding the eyelid open, use a cup or a shower-head to pour a gentle stream of lukewarm water in the eye for 15 minutes (or use sterile eye wash such as contact lens saline rinse).

   Make sure the water is running away from the uncontaminated eye. If your child is wearing contact lenses, remove them, then wash your hands to remove any chemicals.

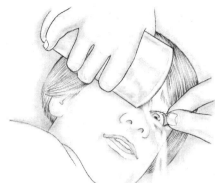

2. Cover the injured eye with a clean dressing, and don't let your child rub his eye.

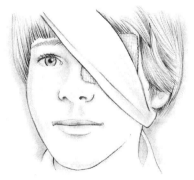

58

Eye Emergencies
Cornea (Eyeball) Scratches

Signs & Symptoms
- Constant blinking of the eyes, light sensitivity, pain.

1. Rinse the eye with a clean solution, preferably saline, or clean water. Have the child blink several times.

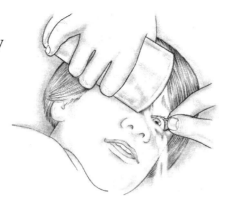

Don'ts
- Don't apply pressure to the cornea (the clear protective outer covering of the eyeball).
- Don't let your child touch her eye.

When to Get Professional Help
- If your child's cornea is scratched, call your doctor or take your child to an emergency facility for a definitive diagnosis and medication, if needed. Corneal scratches or abrasions can become infected.

Eye Emergencies

Eyelid Cuts & Bruises

What You Need to Know

- A black eye occurs when bleeding takes place under the skin around the eye. Though uncommon, this can occur with more serious injuries such as skull fractures and brain injuries.

When to Get Professional Help

- For any cut near the eye, call your doctor or take your child to an emergency facility; a tear duct or nerve may be injured, which requires professional treatment.
- If there are any vision problems (double or blurred vision), severe pain, or bleeding from the eye or nose, the eye should be evaluated professionally.
- If there is blood in the white or colored part of the eye, see your doctor.

1. If the cut is bleeding, apply direct pressure with a clean, dry cloth until the bleeding subsides.

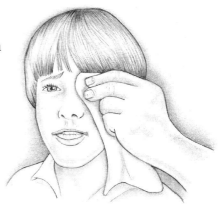

2. Clean the cut with water, cover with a clean dressing, and apply gentle pressure around the eye by placing a cold pack or compress on the dressing (to reduce pain and swelling) for up to 48 hours.

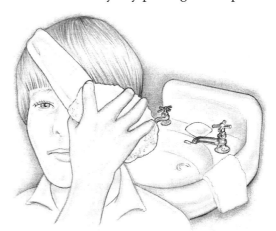

Eye Emergencies
Foreign Objects

1. Wash your hands. Seat your child in a well-lit area. Grasp the top eyelid and pull it out and down over the eye.

   The object may wash out with tears.

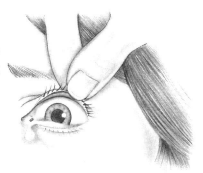

2. Gently depress the lower eyelid and look for the object.

   If you see the object, carefully lift it off with a clean cloth.

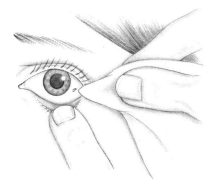

3. Have your child blink, which may force the object out.

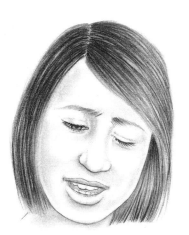

Fainting

What You Need to Know

- Fainting is usually brief and occurs when the blood supply to the brain is temporarily inadequate, causing the child to lose consciousness. The seriousness can range from negligible to severe.

When to Get Professional Help

- If your child does not regain consciousness after 1 minute, call your local emergency number.

Don'ts

- Don't splash water on your child's face, shake him, or use smelling salts.
- Don't give him anything to eat or drink.

Signs & Symptoms

- Paleness, dizziness, sweating, passing out.

1. If your child becomes light-headed, have him lie down for at least 10 to 15 minutes. Elevate his feet above heart level. If he cannot lie down, have him sit down and place his head between his knees.

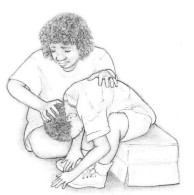

2. Loosen your child's clothing (belts, collars, etc.) and make sure he has sufficient air.

3. If your child loses consciousness, place him on his back and elevate his legs above heart level by 12 inches (30 cm).

   Don't place a pillow under your child's head.

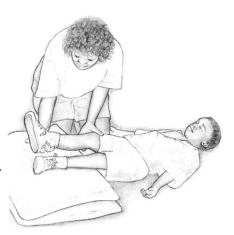

What to Check
- If your child remains unconscious for more than 1 minute, observe breathing and check circulation. If needed, begin CPR:

  If your child is under 1 year old, see page 16, BREATHING/CARDIAC EMERGENCY, For Infant Under 1 Year.

  If your child is 1 to 8 years old, see page 20, BREATHING/CARDIAC EMERGENCY, For Child Age 1–8 Years.

  If your child is over 8 years old, see page 24, BREATHING/CARDIAC EMERGENCY, For Child Over 8 Years.

4. Turn your child's head to the side to prevent him from choking if he vomits.

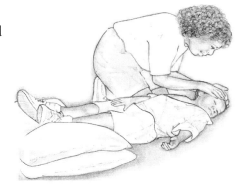

5. Wait 5 to 10 minutes after your child regains consciousness before allowing him to stand or walk.

   If he fell, check for any injuries. If you suspect significant injuries, especially to the head, call your doctor immediately.

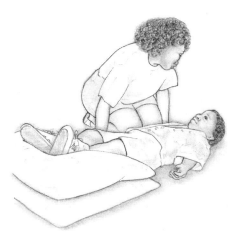

Fever

What You Need to Know

- Many infants and children develop high fevers, even with minor viral illnesses.
- Fevers below 107°F (41.5°C) do not cause brain damage.

When to Get Professional Help

- If an infant younger than 3 or 4 months has a rectal temperature above 100.4°F (38°C), call your doctor. If a child is older than 4 months but younger than 2 years and has a fever higher than 102°F (38.9°C) for more than 1 day, call your doctor. If a child is older than 2 years, call your doctor if the fever is present for more than 3 days.

Don'ts

- Don't use ice water or rubbing alcohol to reduce your child's temperature.
- Don't bundle a feverish child in blankets.
- Don't wake a sleeping child to give her medication or take her temperature; sleep is more important.

1. If your child's temperature is over 102°F (39°C), or if she is uncomfortable, give her pain-relieving tablets or liquid (acetaminophen or ibuprofen).

   Follow the dosage and age guidelines recommended on the package label.

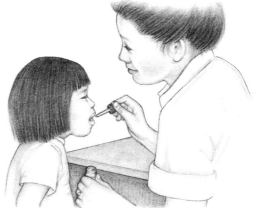

2. Dress your child in light clothing, give her liquids, and keep the room comfortably cool.

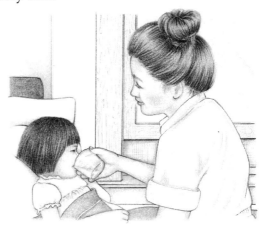

Fractures & Dislocations

Signs & Symptoms
- Pain, swelling, bruising, deformity, limitation of movement, pain on weight bearing.

1. Treat any bleeding with direct pressure.

   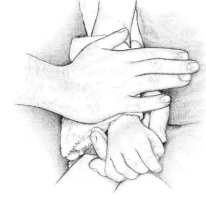

   Turn to page 14—BLEEDING. Cover the wound with a clean dressing.

2. If the injury is to the shoulder or upper arm, immobilize the arm with a triangular cloth sling and tie the sling to the body.

   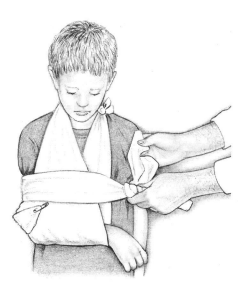

   Turn to page x—HOW TO MAKE A SLING.

What You Need to Know
- A fracture is the cracking, breaking, or buckling of bones; a dislocation is the displacement or slippage of bones from joints.
- Children can have additional risks from fractures because their bones are still growing and the growth plates can be damaged.
- Always immobilize a fractured or dislocated part in the position in which it was found.

What to Check
- If there is heavy bleeding, observe your child for signs of shock. If he becomes dizzy or faint and/or develops pale, cool, clammy skin; rapid, shallow breathing; and a weak, rapid pulse, continue to treat the bleeding and turn to page 79—SHOCK.

When to Get Professional Help

- Call your local emergency number in any of the following circumstances:
  - You suspect an injury to the neck or spine, a severe head injury, or multiple fractures.
  - Your child is unresponsive or not moving.
  - A bone is protruding through the skin.
  - A chest injury is associated with difficulty breathing.
- If your child has a suspected fracture or dislocation, or if even gentle pressure or movement causes pain, call your doctor or take the child to an emergency facility.
- If you suspect a spinal injury or a broken hip, pelvis, or thigh, don't move your child unless absolutely necessary. If you must move him, see Step 5.

3. If the injury is to a limb, immobilize the injured part—in the position in which it was found—with a padded splint.

   Turn to page ix—HOW TO MAKE A SPLINT. The splint should extend both above and below the fracture site. Don't apply the splint too tightly.

   If the injury is to a finger or toe, you can use an adjacent toe or finger as a splint by taping the two digits together.

   If the injury is to a forearm, after splinting it, place the arm in a triangular cloth sling and tie the sling to the body. Turn to page x—HOW TO MAKE A SLING.

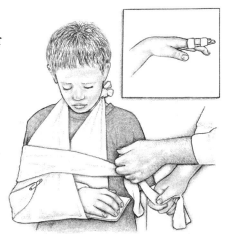

4. If the injury is to the hip, pelvis, or thigh, and you are waiting for an ambulance, immobilize the injured area by placing rolled-up towels, blankets, or clothing between your child's legs. You can also use a large triangular bandage or sling to bind the injured leg to the uninjured leg.

   Don't let your child move his legs.

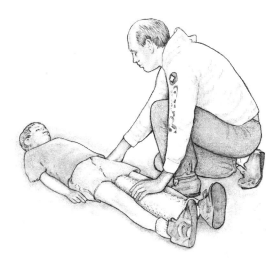

5. If the injury is to the hip, pelvis, or thigh, and you must move your child yourself, immobilize the injured part on a stretcher.

If possible, get several people to help. Use a sturdy board such as an ironing board or another long, flat object that extends from the child's head to his heels. Together, roll his entire body as a unit—keeping the head, neck, and back in a straight line—toward you. Slide the board alongside him. Roll him onto the board, again keeping the head and torso stable. Place rolled-up towels, blankets, or clothing between his legs. Use ropes, belts, tape, or strips of cloth to help hold him in place on the stretcher. Keep him as horizontal as possible when transporting him.

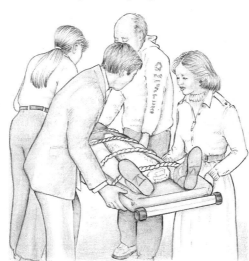

6. Apply a cold compress or cold pack to the injury to reduce pain and limit swelling.

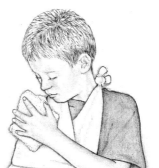

Head Injuries

What You Need to Know

- The signs and symptoms of a head injury may occur immediately or develop slowly over several hours.
- Vomiting as a result of head injury is more common in young children than in older children. Frequent vomiting within a short period, such as more than 1 to 2 times in an hour, may indicate more serious injury.
- A concussion occurs when there is a temporary loss of brain function. Loss of consciousness usually accompanies a concussion.

Signs & Symptoms

- *Minor head injury*: lump or cut on the head, brief period of vomiting, brief loss of consciousness and confusion or double vision, occasionally 1 to 2 hours of drowsiness.
- *Serious head injury*: lump or cut on the head, severe head or facial bleeding, severe headache, unequal pupils, persistent vomiting, extended period of unconsciousness, amnesia, confusion or double vision, drowsiness, slurred speech, convulsions, clear or bloody nasal discharge, bleeding from the ears, black and blue discoloration behind the ears or below the eyes, inability to respond to simple questions or commands or to move uninjured body parts, initial improvement followed by worsening symptoms.

1. Attempt to stop any bleeding by firmly pressing a clean cloth on the wound.

   If the injury is serious, be careful not to move your child's head. If blood soaks through the cloth, don't remove it; you may loosen the clot. Place another cloth over the first one.

2. If the head wound is superficial, wash it with soap and warm water and pat dry.

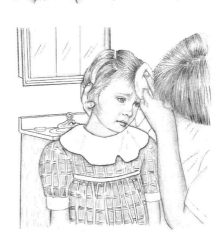

3. If your child is vomiting and you don't suspect a neck or spinal injury, turn her head to the side to prevent her from choking.

   If you suspect a neck or spinal injury, get several people to help, if possible, and together try to roll your child's entire body as a unit—keeping head, neck, and back in a straight line—toward you onto her side.

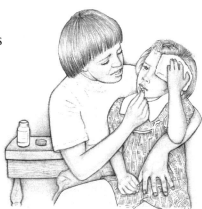

4. If there is swelling and pain, apply a cold compress to the injury and give your child pain-relieving tablets or liquid (acetaminophen or ibuprofen).

   Follow the dosage and age guidelines recommended on the package label.

5. Over the next 12 to 24 hours, observe your child for any signs and symptoms of a serious head injury.

   During the night, wake your child every 1 to 2 hours. If she cannot respond to simple questions or commands, or if vomiting persists, call your doctor or take the child to an emergency facility.

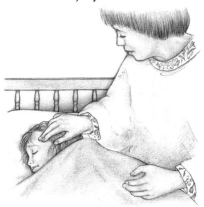

When to Get Professional Help

- If your child shows any of the signs and symptoms of a *serious* head injury, call your local emergency number.
- If your child shows any of the signs or symptoms of a *minor* head injury, call your doctor.

Don'ts

- Don't move your child if you suspect a serious head injury or a spinal injury (see page 80—SPINAL INJURY).
- If your child is wearing a helmet and you suspect a serious head injury, don't remove the helmet.
- Don't wash a head wound that is deep or bleeding profusely.

Heat Emergencies
Heat Cramps/Fatigue/Exhaustion

What to Check
- Take your child's temperature. If your child has a high temperature—102°F to 106°F (39°C to 41°C)—and is not sweating, he may have heat stroke, which can be very serious. Turn immediately to page 71—HEAT EMERGENCIES, Heat Stroke. If his temperature is normal or slightly elevated, follow these first-aid steps.
- If your child is vomiting, turn him on his side to prevent choking.

When to Get Professional Help
- If your child's temperature is high—102°F to 106°F (39°C to 41°C)—call your local emergency number.
- If your child's temperature is above 101°F (38.5°C), or if signs and symptoms last longer than 1 to 2 hours or worsen, call your doctor.

Don'ts
- Don't give your child salt tablets.

Signs & Symptoms
- Fatigue; nausea; cool, moist, and pale skin; dizziness or feeling faint; profuse sweating; rapid, weak pulse; painful involuntary muscle spasms; thirst; dark urine; normal to slightly elevated temperature.

1. Remove your child from sunlight and have him lie down in a cool place.

   Loosen his clothing. Elevate his legs and feet slightly.

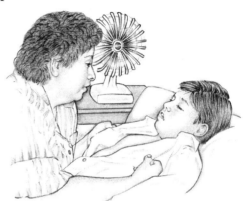

2. Unless your child is vomiting, have him drink cool water or caffeine-free, alcohol-free liquids.

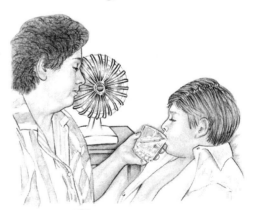

3. Cool your child by sponging or spraying him with cool water and fanning him.

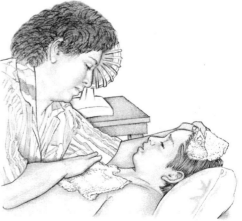

Heat Emergencies

Signs & Symptoms

- Absence of sweating; hot, flushed, dry skin (but it may be moist); headache; dizziness; giddiness; confusion; nausea/vomiting; muscle cramps; bounding or weak-and-rapid pulse; loss of consciousness; high temperature—often 104°F to 106°F (40°C to 41°C).

1. Remove your child from direct sunlight and begin a cool-down procedure.

   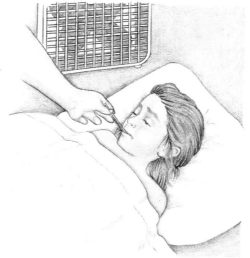

   Lay her down in a cool room in front of a fan or air conditioner and wrap her in damp sheets or spray her with cool water. If the heat stroke is severe or long lasting, apply cold packs on the wrists, ankles, groin, neck, and armpits.

2. If your child is alert enough, have her drink cool water or caffeine-free, alcohol-free liquids.

What You Need to Know

- Heat stroke is the most severe of the heat-related emergencies, often occurring after exercise or heavy work in the heat without sufficient fluid intake. The body's normal mechanisms are unable to deal with the stress caused by the heat. Young children are at increased risk of developing heat stroke.

What to Check

- Observe your child for signs of shock. If she becomes dizzy or faint and/or develops pale, cool, clammy skin; rapid, shallow breathing; and a weak, rapid pulse, turn to page 79—SHOCK.

When to Get Professional Help

- If you suspect heat stroke, call your local emergency number and immediately try to lower your child's body temperature; heat stroke can be very serious.

Don'ts

- Don't give your child medications or stimulants such as caffeinated soft drinks.

Influenza (Flu)

What You Need to Know

- Influenza is a viral respiratory illness that may affect both the upper respiratory tract (nose and throat) and lower respiratory tract (bronchial tubes and lungs). It is more severe than the common cold and strikes almost every child from time to time.
- Symptoms can include nausea, vomiting, and abdominal pain. However, influenza should not be confused with gastroenteritis, sometimes called the "stomach flu," which presents with vomiting and diarrhea as the main symptoms.
- Influenza is highly contagious, spreading by from coughing and sneezing droplets into the air, as well as by touching a contaminated surface or object. It is most frequent in the winter and early spring.
- There are subtypes of influenza, with A and B types responsible for most infections. The terms *avian flu* and *swine flu* or *H1N1* refer to types of influenza that are within the type A and B categories.

Signs & Symptoms

- High fever (103°F to 105°F or 39.4°C to 40.6°C); chills and sweating; muscle aches and pains, especially in the back, arms, and legs; headache; decreased energy; dizziness; dry cough; sore throat; runny or stuffy nose; decreased appetite. In infants, influenza may be accompanied by ear infections, croup, bronchiolitis (small airway infection), and pneumonia.

1. Calm and reassure your child. Try to help her get plenty of rest.

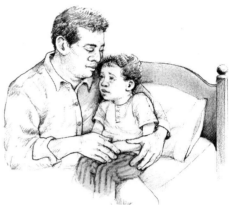

2. If your child is in pain or discomfort and/or has a high fever, give acetaminophen or ibuprofen to help comfort her.

   Follow the dosage and age guidelines recommended on the package label. However, remember that fever is one of the body's way to fight infection, so don't be overaggressive with fever treatment.

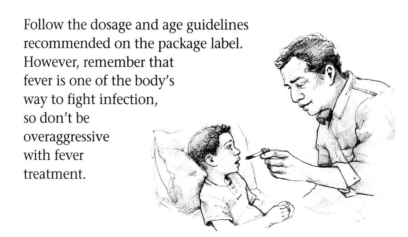

3. Encourage good fluid intake and monitor for signs of dehydration, including decreased urine output, decreased or absent tears, dry lips and mouth, sunken soft spot in infants, and lethargy.

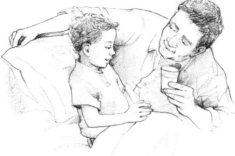

4. Watch for difficulty breathing or a bluish color to her skin. If either occurs, call your local emergency number.

When to Get Professional Help

- If you suspect your child has influenza, contact your doctor early in the illness, as a prescribed antiviral medication may shorten the course of the illness and help prevent the spread of infection to others.
- If your child has underlying health problems, such as heart or lung disease, a weakened immune system, or a malignancy, it is important to have your doctor see your child immediately, as there is increased risk of severe complications from influenza.
- If there are signs of secondary infection such as ear pain, persistent cough or a cough that turns phlegmy, or sharp pain with breathing, have your doctor see your child to check for the need for antibiotics.

Don'ts

- Don't use aspirin or medications containing aspirin to treat influenza.

Nose Emergencies

Bleeding

What You Need to Know

- Dry air, vigorous blowing, nosepicking, and injuries to the nose cause most nosebleeds.

When to Get Professional Help

- If bleeding persists after 15 to 20 minutes of treatment, nosebleeds recur, or blood persistently drains down your child's throat, call your doctor.
- If your child is weak or dizzy, or the bleeding is the result of a blow to the head or a fall, go to an emergency facility.

1. Calm and reassure your child.

   Bleeding will be less severe if she relaxes.

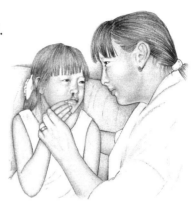

2. Have your child sit upright and lean forward. Pinch her nose shut using your thumb and index finger for at least 5 to 10 minutes, to reduce blood pressure, discourage more bleeding, and help avoid swallowing blood, which can irritate the stomach.

   Don't let her sniff, pick, or blow her nose for several hours. Don't let her bend down, and keep her head higher than her heart. If the bleeding persists or recurs, repeat Step 2.

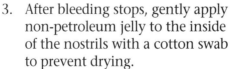

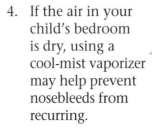

3. After bleeding stops, gently apply non-petroleum jelly to the inside of the nostrils with a cotton swab to prevent drying.

4. If the air in your child's bedroom is dry, using a cool-mist vaporizer may help prevent nosebleeds from recurring.

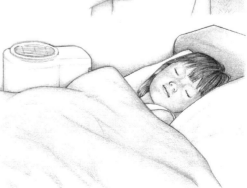

Nose Emergencies
Foreign Objects

Signs & Symptoms
* Bleeding, difficulty breathing, a visible foreign object in the nose, foul-smelling discharge from the nostrils (especially from one nostril).

1. Have your child gently close the unaffected nostril and blow his nose to try to free the object.

2. If the object is not removed and is visible and easy to grasp, try to remove it with a pair of tweezers (round-ended is best).

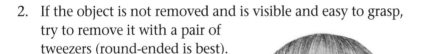

What You Need to Know
* Small children often put foreign objects in their nose.

When to Get Professional Help
* If you can't easily remove the object, call your doctor or take your child to an emergency facility.

Don'ts
* Don't try to remove an object that is not visible and easy to grasp; doing so may push the object farther in and/or damage tissue.
* Don't have your child try to inhale the object.

Nose Emergencies

Injuries

- Bruising under the eyes may occur a day or two after a nose injury.

Signs & Symptoms
- Swelling, redness, pain, bleeding.

1. Calm and reassure your child.

   Bleeding and swelling will be less severe if she relaxes.

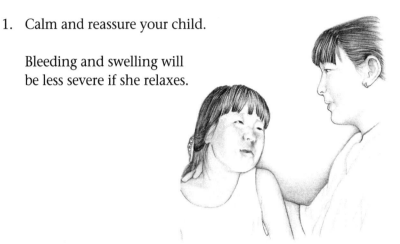

2. Stop bleeding as you would for a nosebleed.

   Turn to page 74—NOSE EMERGENCIES, Bleeding.

3. Apply cold compresses or cold packs to the nose to reduce swelling.

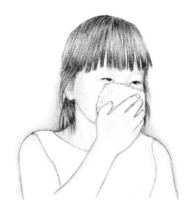

4. Give your child pain-relieving tablets or liquid (acetaminophen or ibuprofen), if needed.

   Follow the dosage and age guidelines recommended on the package label.

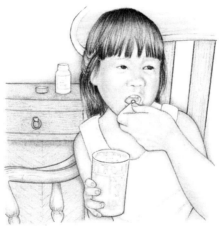

When to Get Professional Help

- If (a) the pain is severe or persists after treatment, (b) the bleeding cannot be controlled or recurs, (c) the nose seems misshapen, or (d) breathing through each nostril separately is difficult, call your doctor.
- Very few nose injuries cause problems requiring immediate professional attention. The doctor may prefer to see your child after the swelling subsides.

Poisoning

What You Need to Know

- Poisoning can be serious, but frequently can be managed at home. Prompt determination of the substance ingested and immediate treatment are essential.
- Medicines, cleaning fluids and products, alcoholic beverages, cosmetics, pesticides, paints and solvents, and houseplants are common causes of poisoning.
- If possible, bring samples of the ingested substance (including any information and first-aid instructions on the product label) and/or the vomit with you to the hospital for analysis.

When to Get Professional Help

- If your child is unconscious and/or has difficulty breathing, call your local emergency number.
- Otherwise, call your local or regional Poison Control Center, doctor, or hospital immediately for instructions.
- Don't induce vomiting unless instructed.

Signs & Symptoms

- Sudden onset of illness or change in behavior, which may take many forms depending on the substance ingested.
- Severe throat pain, difficulty breathing, unexplained nausea or vomiting, burns on the lip or mouth.

1. If your child is conscious, try to determine what he swallowed.

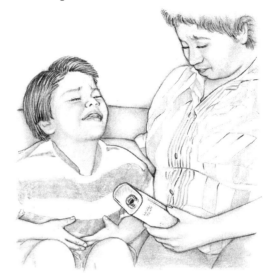

2. Call for help.

3. If your child isn't breathing, begin CPR.

   Follow the CPR directions:

   If your child is under 1 year old, see page 16—BREATHING/ CARDIAC EMERGENCY, For Infant Under 1 Year.

   If your child is 1 to 8 years old, see page 20—BREATHING/ CARDIAC EMERGENCY, For Child Age 1–8 Years.

   If your child is over 8 years old, see page 24—BREATHING/ CARDIAC EMERGENCY, For Child Over 8 Years.

Shock

Signs & Symptoms
- Pale or gray, cool, clammy skin; dizziness/faintness; eyes that are staring or lack luster; thirst; nausea/vomiting; rapid, shallow breathing; weak, rapid pulse; low blood pressure.
- Unconsciousness might or might not occur.

1. Check your child's ABC (airway, breathing, and circulation). If your child is conscious and doesn't have a head or chest injury with difficulty breathing, place her on her back and elevate her feet 12 inches (30 cm).

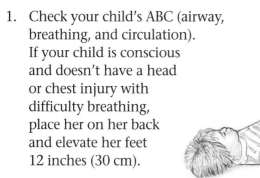

2. Loosen tight clothing to keep your child comfortable and cover her with a blanket or jacket to keep her warm.

   Assess for other injuries, bleeding, or fractures and treat these appropriately.

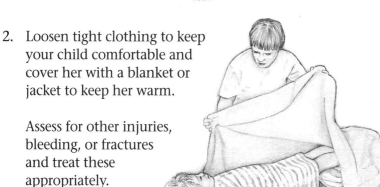

3. If your child isn't breathing, begin CPR.

   Follow the CPR directions:

   If your child is under 1 year old, see page 16—BREATHING/CARDIAC EMERGENCY, For Infant Under 1 Year.

   If your child is 1 to 8 years old, see page 20—BREATHING/CARDIAC EMERGENCY, For Child Age 1–8 Years.

   If your child is over 8 years old, see page 24—BREATHING/CARDIAC EMERGENCY, For Child Over 8 Years.

What You Need to Know
- Shock may result from injuries with extensive blood loss, a severe allergic reaction, a serious infection, poisoning, severe burns, heat stroke, or heart disease.
- When in shock, the body organs do not get enough oxygen or blood.
- If shock results from blood loss, stop the bleeding before treating the shock.

Don'ts
- If you suspect spinal injury, don't move your child.
- Don't give your child anything to eat or drink, even if she complains of thirst.

When to Get Professional Help
- If you suspect shock, call your local emergency number. Shock requires immediate treatment to prevent damage to vital organs and tissues.

Spinal Injury

What You Need to Know

- Neck and back injuries need to be taken seriously because of the risk of paralysis and even death. Moving the child can cause further damage to spinal cord nerves.
- Any accidents that involve landing on the head—such as from diving, bike and car injuries, or contact sports—or accidents with a major blow to the head, neck, or chest can result in spinal injuries.

Signs & Symptoms

- Stiff neck, severe pain in the neck area, headache, head held in unusual position, weakness, numbness, tingling or inability to move the extremities, difficulty standing or walking, loss of bowel or bladder control, shock, and the signs associated with a serious head injury (turn to page 68—HEAD INJURIES).

1. If your child is unconscious, check for breathing.

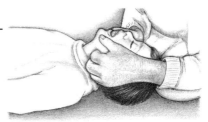

   Without tilting your child's head back or moving or lifting the neck or head, pull the jaw forward to open the airway. Make sure the tongue is not obstructing the airway. Look, listen, and feel for breathing.

   If he is breathing, go to Step 3.

2. If your child isn't breathing, begin CPR.

   Follow the CPR directions:

   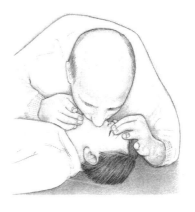

   If your child is under 1 year old, see page 16—BREATHING/CARDIAC EMERGENCY, For Infant Under 1 Year.

   If your child is 1 to 8 years old, see page 20—BREATHING/CARDIAC EMERGENCY, For Child Age 1–8 Years.

   If your child is over 8 years old, see page 24—BREATHING/CARDIAC EMERGENCY, For Child Over 8 Years.

   When he resumes regular breathing, go to Step 3. Continue to observe breathing and check the pulse.

3. Immobilize your child's head and torso in the position found.

   Place rolled-up towels, clothing, or blankets around his head, neck, and torso. If your child is on his back, slide a pad or small towel under his neck without moving his head. Make sure his collar is loose. Keep supports in place with heavy objects such as books or stones. If possible, tape his forehead as shown.

   If emergency personnel are on the way, no further treatment is needed.

4. If you must move your child, get several people to help. Do not try to move him alone.

   Use a sturdy support, such as an ironing board or a plank, as a stretcher. Together, roll your child's entire body as a unit—keeping head, neck, and back in a straight line— toward you. Slide the board alongside the child. Roll him onto the board, keeping the head and torso stable.

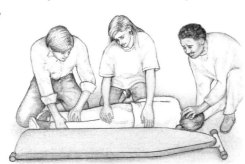

5. Immobilize your child's head and torso in the position found.

   Place rolled-up towels, clothing, or blankets around his head and torso. Use ropes, belts, tape, or strips of cloth to hold him in place on the stretcher. Carry the stretcher as horizontally as possible.

When to Get Professional Help
- Call your local emergency number immediately for any back or neck injury, in addition to following these first-aid steps.

Don'ts
- Don't bend, twist, or lift your child's head or body.
- Don't attempt to move your child before medical help arrives. If he must be moved, see Steps 4 and 5.
- If your child is wearing a helmet, don't remove it.

Sprains & Strains

When to Get Professional Help

- If (a) the pain or swelling is severe, (b) your child's ability to move the affected area is limited, (c) a bone is deformed and possibly broken, (d) there are signs of infection, including the area feeling hot or your child has a fever, (e) the affected area feels numb, (f) your child felt a pop or tear at the time of injury, (g) the injured area remains painful after 48 hours, or (h) your child is unable to apply pressure to the injured area after 48 hours, call your doctor.

Signs & Symptoms

- Pain, swelling, stiffness, limitation of joint movement, bruising.

1. Have your child rest in a comfortable position.

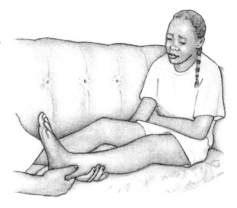

2. If possible, elevate the injured area above heart level to slow blood flow and reduce swelling. Continue elevation for 24 to 48 hours after the injury.

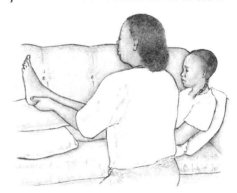

3. Apply a cold compress to the injured area for 10 to 15 minutes to reduce swelling and pain.

If swelling persists, reapply the cold compress every 20 to 30 minutes until the swelling decreases. If the injury is new and requires professional help, apply ice or a cold compress during the ride to your doctor or emergency center.

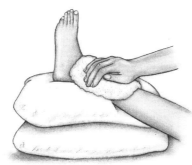

4. Give your child pain-relieving tablets or liquid (acetaminophen or ibuprofen), if needed.

Follow the dosage and age guidelines recommended on the package label.

What You Need to Know

- A *sprain* is the tearing and/or stretching of a ligament; they're usually caused by falling, twisting, or getting hit in the affected area. A *strain* is the tearing and/or stretching of muscle fibers or tendons.
- Typical areas affected are fingers, wrists, ankles, knees, and foot arches.
- If you suspect a fracture, turn to page 65—FRACTURES & DISLOCATIONS.

Continue to the next page

5. If your child has an injury to the leg, ankle, or knee, gently wrap the affected area with an elastic bandage firmly but not tightly.

    You may want to use a soft splint or pillow to help keep the area immobilized.

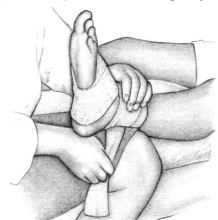

6. If your child has an injury to the shoulder, elbow, or wrist, immobilize the arm with a triangular cloth sling and tie the sling to the body.

    Turn to page x—HOW TO MAKE A SLING.

7. After 48 hours, if pain and swelling have decreased, have your child try to move the affected joint in all directions.

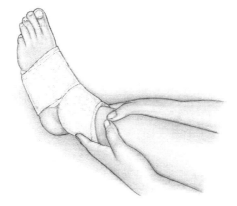

8. Keep pressure off the injured area until the pain subsides, usually 7 to 10 days for mild sprains and strains and 4 to 6 weeks for severe sprains and strains.

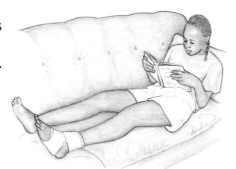

Parents' Emergency Information Page

LOCAL EMERGENCY PHONE: _____

DOCTOR OR CLINIC:

Name _____

Phone _____

Address _____

HOSPITAL:

Name _____

Phone _____

Address _____

Directions to Hospital _____

POISON CONTROL CENTER: _____

FIRE: _____

POLICE: _____

ANIMAL CONTROL OR VETERINARIAN: _____

NEIGHBOR OR RELATIVE:

Name _____ Phone _____

Name _____ Phone _____

Name _____ Phone _____

Name _____ Phone _____

MOTHER: Work_____ Cell_____

FATHER: Work_____ Cell_____